T0383020

THE OFFICIAL
MIND DIET

ALSO BY DR. MARTHA CLARE MORRIS

Diet for the MIND:
The Latest Science on What to Eat to
Prevent Alzheimer's and Cognitive Decline

· THE OFFICIAL ·

MIND DIET

A Scientifically Based Program to
Lose Weight and Prevent Alzheimer's Disease

Dr. Martha Clare Morris

with Laura Morris and Jennifer Ventrelle

Little, Brown Spark
New York   Boston   London

Little, Brown Spark
Hachette Book Group
1290 Avenue of the Americas, New York, NY 10104
littlebrownspark.com

First Edition: December 2023

Little, Brown Spark is an imprint of Little, Brown and Company, a division of Hachette Book Group, Inc. The Little, Brown Spark name and logo are trademarks of Hachette Book Group, Inc.

The publisher is not responsible for websites (or their content) that are not owned by the publisher.

The Hachette Speakers Bureau provides a wide range of authors for speaking events. To find out more, go to hachettespeakersbureau.com or email HachetteSpeakers@hbgusa.com.

Little, Brown and Company books may be purchased in bulk for business, educational, or promotional use. For information, please contact your local bookseller or the Hachette Book Group Special Markets Department at special.markets@hbgusa.com.

Text illustrations by iStockphoto

ISBN 9780316441186
LCCN 2023942073

Printing 3, 2024

LSC-C

Printed in the United States of America

In loving memory of Dr. Martha Clare Morris,
a pioneer in the field of nutrition and dementia,
who believed that all contributions, whether big
or small, were important and valuable.
Alone we can accomplish so little;
together we can accomplish so much.

Contents

INTRODUCTION: The Dinner Table 3

PART I
THE RESEARCH BEHIND THE MIND DIET

CHAPTER 1: The Problem of Alzheimer's Disease — and
Its Solution? 13

CHAPTER 2: The Research on Nutrients for the Brain 18

CHAPTER 3: The MIND Diet and Its Evidence for
Protection against Neurodegenerative Diseases 26

CHAPTER 4: The MIND Diet Intervention to Prevent
Alzheimer's Disease 30

CHAPTER 5: The Loss of a Great Leader 33

CHAPTER 6: Exciting New Research on the MIND Diet 38

PART II
FOODS FOR BRAIN HEALTH

CHAPTER 7: NeverMIND the Diet 47

CHAPTER 8: Vegetables (Plural) and Fruit (Singular) 60

CHAPTER 9: Unsaturated Fats: Extra-Virgin Olive Oil, Nuts,
and Seeds 76

CHAPTER 10: Proteins: Fish, Seafood, and Poultry 88

CHAPTER 11: Carbohydrates: Whole Grains, Beans,
and Legumes 99

Contents

CHAPTER 12: Wine in Moderation — 113

CHAPTER 13: Saturated Fats: Red Meat, Butter, Cheese, Fried Foods, and Sweets — 117

CHAPTER 14: MIND Diet FAQs: Lessons Learned from the Field — 124

PART III
YOUR MIND DIET TOOLBOX FOR SUCCESS

CHAPTER 15: The Essential Tools — 131

CHAPTER 16: Tools for Weight Loss — 168

CHAPTER 17: Your MINDful Life — 182

PART IV
THE OFFICIAL MIND DIET 6-WEEK PROGRAM

CHAPTER 18: 6 Weeks to a Healthy MIND — 201

PART V
THE MIND DIET RECIPES

CHAPTER 19: Your Kitchen, Your Home — 237

CHAPTER 20: Breakfast — 240

CHAPTER 21: Main Meals — 254

CHAPTER 22: Sides, Salads, and Snacks — 287

CHAPTER 23: Sweets — 303

CHAPTER 24: Sauces and Toppers — 314

Acknowledgments — 323

Notes — 327

Appendix: The MIND Diet Program at a Glance and Sample Meal Plan — 337

Index — 348

THE OFFICIAL
MIND DIET

Introduction:
The Dinner Table

by Laura Morris

"Some people might look at what I do and wonder how I could love it—so much of it is statistics and numbers and reading and writing very technical documents. My kids look at me like I must be crazy the way I can get positively giddy about my data. My passion drives me to pursue the never-ending circle of questions and answers in my scientific field, and to do it in the face of continual criticism and rejection that make up the scientific world. There are as many theories and interpretations of the same data as there are scientists. Our limitations as human beings inhibit our understanding of truth. I view science as a great onion in which we peel back one layer after another. Each layer gives us another piece of understanding about the world we live in, but a view that may change when we peel back the next layer, the next discovery. This can cause much frustration when the science world seems to flip-flop. But these flip-flops are a necessary by-product of the process. As we peel off the layers of the onion, we may never get to the ultimate truth of our worlds even though we increase our understanding. Appreciation and enjoyment of the process of seeking truth must be what it is all about. And perhaps what life itself is all about. The journey and the love and the faith in our quest are the very heart of happiness and joy."

— *Dr. Martha Clare Morris*

The dinner table was a sacred place in our home. Some of my earliest memories are of my family gathered around, my mom smiling as she usually did, dressed to the nines with her hair in bouncy blonde curls. My father, always a grand presence in his jeans and smoking his pipe, laughing at something while enthusiastically smacking his knee. My brother, sister, and I recounting what happened at school. No matter how hard, frustrating, uplifting, or triumphant the day may have been, the five of us always drifted to this special spot to share our experiences, to listen, and to be together. Dinnertime was our sanctuary, our daily meditation for our souls. If someone was running late, we would all wait at the table until that person got home. And once we started our meal, we weren't in a hurry to finish—we always lingered until everyone shared what they had been doing that day. Oftentimes, friends, neighbors, and co-workers were invited to scooch in a chair and fill their plate. My parents just had a way of making everyone feel welcome.

The dinner table also became a classroom of sorts. Growing up a child of a nutritional epidemiologist is a unique experience (if you know, you know!). Every meal, food, and nutrient that we ate was an opportunity to talk about the vast and abundant nutritional compounds we were ingesting. My mother never missed the chance to share her knowledge with us, to instill an appreciation for the magic of food as medicine. The funny thing is, although my siblings and I were immersed in our own childhood or adolescent dramas, we couldn't help but catch a bit of the passion she had about the biochemical reactions happening in our bodies when we ate a certain food. It was like she was telling tales about the discovery of the moon.

I can remember when I was 9 years old and she was reading her thesis on fish oil and hypertension aloud to me. It was well over a hundred pages, and she was so excited to share all the information she had gathered. It was one of the few times I couldn't fake being excited; it was just too long. Quite honestly, I just wanted to get back to playing with my dolls. But what I would never forget was her excitement, her eyes sparkling with endless possibilities for what further research would reveal. Little did I know this was just the beginning of a journey I would share with her for the next 30 years.

My mother's passion for nutrition began when she first became pregnant with my older sister, Clare, and from there she was determined to provide all her babies with the very best nutrients. She also began her training in epidemiology around that time and became fiercely adamant about teaching her children how to choose foods with high nutrient density, full of protective antioxidant "soldiers" and free radical–fighting "captains" to help our bodies be as capable as they can be. As her education advanced, the more her understanding of the role food played in health became a central theme to our lives.

Even when I was a small child, I was informed of not just what but *why* I was eating certain foods. I knew that the spinach I was eating was supplying me not only with fiber and folic acid but also with a good dose of polyphenolic compounds. These compounds provided the plant with pigment to protect it from the damaging rays of the sun, so when I ate spinach, I knew I was getting those protective benefits. I also knew that putting a drizzle of olive oil on my vegetables was aiding in the absorption of all the fat-soluble vitamins I was consuming, all while giving me a dose of healthy fats. This all may seem a little over-the-top, and in a way it was. But I should point out that we didn't always eat from the healthy food list. We had our pizza nights, our milkshake runs, or my dad's favorite (usually when my mom was out of town for work), a slab of ribs with french fries. We loved these treats, yet we also knew that if we ate too many of these high-fat foods, they might affect our bodies' ability to perform optimally, or, if eaten frequently, they could cause diseases over time. In our home, eating wasn't about restriction, discipline, or vanity, but rather about appreciating the bounty of nutrients we were getting.

Although the subject of nutrition was fascinating to Mom, it was her research on how the nutrients we eat play a role in brain health that became her obsession. For the longest time, Alzheimer's disease was thought to be mostly genetic. When my mother entered the field of epidemiology in the early nineties and became a "disease detective," she focused particularly on this question of whether nutrients affected the brain, something that nobody else was studying at the time. The more her research revealed a link between food and the way the brain ages, the more consumed she became with her investigation. She was 5 years into her research when her mother-in-law was diagnosed with Alzheimer's, and her work took on a new importance. It had turned into a mission.

I remember when I was 14 years old, my dad told me, "Gramma is getting lost when she goes out for walks." I knew enough about dementia from my mother's work to know that this was not good, and that she would most likely not get better. This was the first time I felt the "beginning of the end" of a loved one's life. What I didn't know was how utterly helpless and devasting it would be to watch my beloved grandmother succumb to Alzheimer's. She had always been the queen bee: mother of seven children, grandmother to fifteen, and the ultimate warrior of life, discipline, wit, and intelligence. We watched as she slowly drifted away—turning into someone we did not recognize. She had been the one person everyone could go to for the hard truth, a pep talk, and infinite wisdom. Seeing her slip away and lose those attributes was heartbreaking for the whole family. The only thing we could do was try to take care of her as she had taken care of us. My grandmother died from Alzheimer's disease 10 years after her symptoms started, at 84 years old.

My grandmother was one of Mom's heroes. Seeing her mother-in-law's decline, being involved in her support and care, and feeling how taxing it was on the family gave her a different lens through which to view Alzheimer's disease. Now it wasn't just about data analysis, brain pathology, and cognitive tests. She had witnessed how Alzheimer's ravages the part of the brain that connects us to our soul—our memories, values, and personality. Although I believe my mom would have worked just as hard for preventative treatments for dementia if she had not experienced this personal loss, it certainly gave her work new meaning and purpose.

Years after my grandmother died, Dr. Martha Clare Morris became known as one of the top researchers in the world studying the link between nutrition and dementia. She spent her career collaborating with other internationally renowned scientists, working together toward a better understanding of nutrients' effects on the brain. Her 25 years of studying dietary patterns, analyzing data from around the world, and looking at brain pathology produced the MIND (Mediterranean-DASH Intervention for Neurodegenerative Delay) Diet.

HOW THIS BOOK EVOLVED

The MIND diet was published in 2015 in the journal *Alzheimer's & Dementia*.[1] The study enlisted volunteers already participating in Rush University's Memory and Aging Project (MAP) and examined their dietary intake from 2004 to 2013. The MAP study looked at dietary patterns of 923 volunteers and created a score based on adherence to the MIND diet. The study showed that the MIND diet reduced the risk of Alzheimer's disease by 53 percent in those who followed the diet rigorously, and by around 35 percent in those who followed it moderately well. The publication took the science community by storm. Since then, the MIND diet has consistently ranked among the top 10 diets for 7 consecutive years by *U.S. News & World Report*[2] and was deemed to have not only long-term cognitive benefits but cardiovascular benefits as well. In 2016, my mother and her colleagues secured funding from the National Institutes of Health (NIH) to do the first-ever randomized dietary intervention trial for dementia, a study that was projected to be completed in 2021.

Sadly, Mom isn't here to see the results of the trial and take that next step forward with her research. In February 2020, my mother, at the pinnacle of her career, passed away at the age of 64 from a rare cancer. Although nothing can fill the void she has left, I take comfort in knowing her contributions to the fields of nutrition and brain health will have long-lasting impact on the world.

My mother certainly influenced my own professional path. The foundation of health that she ingrained in me eventually steered me toward a career in personal training and nutrition consulting, where I worked directly with people to help them on their own journeys to better health. I then pursued a culinary degree to expand my knowledge of all things nourishment.

During a formative period in my professional life, I worked at Rush University with Dr. Christy Tangney, a brilliant nutritionist and colleague of my mother's, in the clinical nutrition department. There, I was lucky enough to meet one of Rush's premier dietitians, Jennifer Ventrelle, when we were working together on a clinical trial on nutritional interventions for women with breast cancer. I was immediately drawn to Jen because of her passion, determination, and commitment to educating her patients on bettering their lives through nutrition and wellness. She was an excellent team player and collaborator in all aspects of her work — clearly wanting nothing more than to make a difference in the lives of her patients.

In 2016, when my mother was putting together her team to conduct the MIND diet trial, she asked me what I thought of Jen as a possible leader on the study. Without hesitation I told her she would not find anyone better. I jokingly told her that Jen was a brunette version of herself — an optimistic, fierce go-getter with an unsurpassed work ethic. Months into working with Jen, my mother called to tell me I was absolutely spot-on about her.

In 2017, a year after setting up the MIND diet trial, my mother completed her first book, *Diet for the MIND: The Latest Science on What to Eat to Prevent Alzheimer's and Cognitive Decline,*[3] which focused on the scientific evidence of the link between nutrition and brain health. Her intention was to come out with a second book that would highlight the MIND diet and concentrate more on a lifestyle plan to show people exactly how to benefit from her research. After my mom died, I knew I wanted no one else but Jen to help complete the program for this book and provide the most up-to-date research on cognitive health. I am honored that Jen has refined the MIND diet program for our readers. This book is the result, combining Jen's expertise with my mother's scientific mission, as well as my own passion for preparing delicious and nutritious foods. It's been a labor of love.

While it's certainly a privilege to share my mother's professional legacy, it's my hope that her personal legacy will serve as inspiration as well. She spent each day living fully and healthfully, always with a big, loving smile. She usually greeted the dawn with an alarming amount of energy and would wake us singing, "Rise and shine like the stars that you are!" She worked out every morning and then would walk to the train to get to work because she liked the fresh air, even on the coldest winter days in Chicago. In the evening, she would often call one of her many close friends to connect. She ended her day with journaling—most often about what was going well with work and why, or what challenges she was facing and what she could do to overcome them. The search for growth—and the discipline required for that growth—brought her great meaning and joy. Her daily lifestyle practices were the foundation of her life and now are a part of mine. When life gets hard or exhausting, I turn to the medicine of food, movement, sleep, and human connection. I really listen to what my body and mind need to power through difficult times. So, in a way, she's with me every day.

My mother operated on all cylinders—and there were lots of them! But no matter how busy she was, she always made time for gathering around that dinner table, nourishing herself and her family with both food and fellowship. I hope you are inspired by her life and research and find ways to incorporate the MIND diet foods into your favorite recipes. But most important, my wish is that you've found your own dinner table surrounded by good friends, family, laughter, and nutritious foods, to move your life forward with joy, purpose, and love.

PART I

THE RESEARCH BEHIND THE MIND DIET

"I love what I do. I get caught up in the whole scientific process—obsessing over every step: assembling the right team, training, and motivating the team to provide unbiased, precise data; analyzing every possible angle of the data in an attempt to discern the truth; and writing draft after draft of my scientific manuscripts until I have clearly and concisely communicated the most important points. This is the never-ending cyclical process, so I am pretty much in a constant state of obsession. The truth about science is that we never do know the truth and there is rarely a visible end product. So having a passion for the process keeps us searching for understanding about the universe. It is an exercise that gives meaning to my life."

—*Dr. Martha Clare Morris*

CHAPTER 1

The Problem of Alzheimer's Disease — and Its Solution?

By Dr. Martha Clare Morris and Laura Morris

It is hard to mention Alzheimer's disease without hearing about a direct personal experience someone has had with it. This is not surprising, because an estimated 6.2 million Americans (one in nine people aged 65 and older) suffer from this affliction.[1] Between the years 2000 and 2019, deaths from Alzheimer's disease increased 145 percent, and it's now the seventh leading cause of death in the United States. Not only is this alarming, but it's projected that 12.7 million people will have Alzheimer's dementia by 2050. But what *is* Alzheimer's disease and how is it different from general cognitive decline and dementia?

DIAGNOSING DEMENTIA

Let's start by looking at the way the brain ages. There are many different types of thinking we use to get through our day. For example,

---

Note from Laura Morris: I've compiled chapters 1–4 from my mother's notes. For purposes of clarity, I've kept them in her voice. Registered dietitian Jennifer Ventrelle and nutritionist Dr. Christy Tangney confirmed all details regarding scientific data.

we store memories that help us manage basic tasks, such as brushing our teeth and getting dressed. We also have reasoning skills, which we use to figure out how to reach a destination, for example. There's also the speed at which we can process different pieces of information to then make decisions, for instance when we are taking a math test or carrying on a conversation. Most of us experience some decline in cognitive abilities as we get older. Just as with our muscles, there is a gradual decline in the normal functioning of our brains. Our ability to problem-solve or to retrieve words may slow down. Forgetting a person's name is a temporary loss that ordinarily does not affect one's day-to-day functions. These changes are normal with the aging brain. We call this *cognitive decline*.

Mild cognitive impairment (MCI) is when people experience a significant decline in their usual cognitive abilities, such as speed of cognitive processing or memory, but not to the extent that it interferes with performance of their daily activities. People with MCI are still able to take care of their usual responsibilities, and even though they are at an increased risk of developing dementia, many never present with the disease. However, 10 to 15 percent of people with MCI will go on to develop Alzheimer's disease.

Then there is *dementia*, a broad term for the decline in cognitive abilities that is severe enough to interfere with daily life. This could mean forgetting how to use a can opener or not being able to balance a checkbook. Under the umbrella of "dementia" are several different types, Alzheimer's disease being the most common form. The second most common is *vascular dementia*, which is caused by strokes and conditions involving the cardiovascular system. Vascular dementia is more likely to present as an abrupt decrease in cognitive abilities, which is a lot different from the slow, progressive decline that we see with Alzheimer's. Symptoms like the inability to use language appropriately can appear in just a few days. The third common type of dementia is *Lewy body dementia*. This occurs when protein deposits, called Lewy bodies, accumulate in the neurons of the brain, causing those neurons to die. People with Lewy body dementia might have visual hallucinations and changes in alertness and attention. Some symptoms, like rigid muscles, slow movement, walking difficulty, and tremors, can mimic those of Parkinson's disease.

Keep in mind that a number of treatable conditions can cause symptoms similar to those of dementia, such as depression, drug use and drug interactions, thyroid issues, alcohol abuse, dehydration, and vitamin deficiencies. It's important to see a neurologist if you are having trouble with your thinking abilities so you can be properly evaluated for these conditions.

A CLOSER LOOK AT ALZHEIMER'S DISEASE

As mentioned, the most common type of dementia is Alzheimer's disease, where one loses more and more cognitive abilities over time. For a diagnosis of Alzheimer's, a patient must have memory loss *plus one other loss* in cognitive ability, perhaps the ability to solve problems. The diagnosis should be made by a trained clinician in the area of cognition in combination with a neurological exam, medical history, and specialized cognitive testing. There is an exponential increase in prevalence of Alzheimer's with older age. It affects about 5 percent of people aged 65 to 74, 13 percent of those 75 to 84, and about 33 percent of those 85 and older.[2]

Alzheimer's usually starts in the hippocampus, the part of the brain that controls the ability to learn new tasks and form new memories. So typical early symptoms are difficulty recalling newly acquired information and asking for the same information again and again.

Inside the brain of a person with Alzheimer's are two types of common pathology: *beta amyloid plaques* and *neurofibrillary tangles*. We all have plaques and tangles as we age, but it is the amount of them that indicates signs of Alzheimer's disease.

Plaques form when an abnormal protein called beta amyloid starts to accumulate on the outside of the nerve cells or neurons. Think of these plaques as barnacles covering rocks. When they build up in the brain, they interfere with the neurons' ability to communicate with one another to produce a memory or complete a task. Eventually the neurons will die, and the brain tissue will atrophy.

Neurofibrillary tangles happen when the inside of the neuron has tangled nerve filaments, making it difficult for the neuron to function the way it's meant to. Think of these filaments as tubes that transport nutrients within the cell. *Tau*, one of the proteins inside the brain, is an essential component of these nerve filaments. When it gets damaged, it collapses and twists into tangles, kind of like a big knot in your hair. This leads to neuron loss and brain atrophy, which is considerable in the later stages of Alzheimer's.

REASONS FOR HOPE

Of course, our fears about getting Alzheimer's disease are well founded. It's a painful illness—not just for the person afflicted but also for loved ones and caregivers. Though we've come so far in our understanding of the causes and treatment of heart disease and cancer (two of the biggest killers in our society), treatments for Alzheimer's are largely ineffective and the disease remains incurable.

There has long been an assumption that Alzheimer's disease is genetic, and therefore you have no control over whether you get it or not. However, research from the past 35 years has shown there's a lot we can do to reduce the risk. Much of it boils down to lifestyle factors.

In a nutshell, what is good for your heart is also good for your brain. Each of the major risk factors for cardiovascular diseases—high blood pressure, abnormal cholesterol levels, obesity, and diabetes—are also risk factors for developing dementia and cognitive decline. This is crucial information, because it means when you work to prevent cardiovascular disease, you are concurrently working to ward off Alzheimer's and other dementias. So be sure to get exercise, reduce stress, and manage your blood pressure and cholesterol levels. There's much that we can control in our lifestyles to help us age more healthfully and give us a greater chance at preventing or delaying dementia—and one of the biggest prevention factors is what you put in your body.

I am more optimistic now than I've ever been that we have real weapons in our arsenal for fighting this awful disease now that we better understand some of the preventive factors. And I'm even more enthusiastic that I can offer a path that may greatly reduce your risk of Alzheimer's disease: the MIND diet.

CHAPTER 2

The Research on Nutrients
for the Brain

I am an epidemiologist, which means I study disease in populations. As a scientific investigator, I search for the cause of the disease, identify those who are at risk, and determine how to control, stop, or prevent the disease. My personal expertise is in evaluating the strengths and weaknesses of the way a study is designed, particularly studies on nutrition and the brain. I should emphasize that my recommendations do not stem from the direct evaluation and treatment of patients, in the way a medical doctor would look at things. Nor are they gathered from theories found in a petri dish and then compared to the complex human body in a state of disease. Instead, my mastery is in providing a thorough review of the scientific literature, in filtering out the biased and unreliable studies. Therefore, every nutrient and food that I recommend for brain health and longevity has been rigorously studied and is based on the strongest scientific evidence available.

I trained and received my doctorate degree from the Harvard School of Public Health (renamed the Harvard T. H. Chan School of Public Health), where I had the great fortune to study with one of the best nutritional epidemiologists in the world, Dr. Walter Willett. He has made tremendous contributions to our understanding of the role nutrients play in disease and human health. Not only was Dr. Willett a great mentor to me on how to conduct nutritional investigations, but he was also instrumental in showing me the importance of collaboration and integrity within the scientific community.

When I started my career as an assistant professor at Rush University in Chicago in 1993, it was with a group that was embarking on a large study on the south side of Chicago, called the Chicago Health and Aging Project (CHAP), that focused on the risk factors that contribute to Alzheimer's disease.[1] This study fully and comprehensively evaluated people's lifestyle behaviors and health conditions and followed them over time to track cognitive changes.

At the time, few in the scientific community, including the CHAP study investigators, were looking at diet. There was a bias that presumed diet couldn't possibly have anything to do with the brain—dementia in particular. With my training in nutritional investigations, I had the opportunity to add the study of nutrients to CHAP as a possible component of the risk factors of Alzheimer's disease. Initially, it was hard to get funding, but after many attempts, I received a grant in 1996 to add diet as a possible component. In this large study of more than 10,000 older people, we were able to follow them for more than 20 years. My team and I collected data on their diets, and then related it to what kinds of nutrients they were getting, and how that impacted their brain. We could then evaluate their change in cognitive ability with age over time and the development of Alzheimer's. The CHAP study was pivotal to the start of examining diet in relation to dementia.[2]

Then in 1997, I became involved in another large study at Rush University led by Dr. David Bennett, specifically on this topic, which was called the Memory and Aging Project (MAP).[3] Here we recruited over 1,800 volunteers from retirement communities all over Chicago. Participants were evaluated annually in a 3-hour examination, where we tested for neurological conditions, evaluated cognitive abilities with 20 cognitive tests, and collected information on dietary intake. Participants also agreed to donate their brains after they died, which was especially critical, as we could evaluate what had happened in their brains and could compare that to their diet patterns. The CHAP and MAP studies were both funded by the National Institutes of Health (NIH) and the Alzheimer's Association, and generated numerous findings of dietary links to diseases in the brain like dementia. From those two major studies, we uncovered key nutrients that were shown to have both strong and moderate associations for brain protection.

WHAT WE FOUND: THE "ESSENTIALS"

After reviewing the evidence, we found these nutrients to have the biggest effect on brain health:

1. **Vitamin E**

   Vitamin E is one of the primary fat-soluble antioxidant nutrients found in the brain. The alpha tocopherol form of vitamin E has its own transport protein that delivers itself directly to the brain. Vitamin E resides within the neuron cell membrane, so it can snatch up damaging free-radical molecules as they are generated, providing immediate protection to the neurons against oxidative damage, as well as the development of the amyloid plaques that define Alzheimer's.

   In the MAP study, we measured vitamin E in the brain and found that participants who had higher levels had fewer plaques and tangles than those with lower levels.[4] Other studies have measured vitamin E levels in the blood and concluded that those with high vitamin E blood levels have slower cognitive decline and less risk of developing Alzheimer's disease.[5]

   What about vitamin E supplements? The truth is, we just do not have enough studies to know the answer to this question. The standard amount of vitamin E provided by supplements is either 400 or 800 IU — far higher than what we consume through food, which is around 22 IU. That's a huge difference! Some studies in which people were given high-dose supplements (for example, 400 IU) found that the higher the dose of alpha tocopherol, the lower the levels of gamma tocopherol. Keep in mind that gamma tocopherol is an anti-inflammatory and antioxidant compound as well. So when we put a single nutrient in a supplement, we don't really know what we are doing to the body. I encourage you to improve your diet rather than take supplements.

2. DHA (Docosahexaenoic Acid)

DHA is a type of omega-3 fatty acid that is found in cold-water fish like salmon and tuna. It is an important component that forms the cell membranes of neurons in the brain and has been found to be key for synaptic connections. There's been quite a bit of research linking omega-3 fatty acids to neurocognitive development in the fetus and in the first years of life, which then prompted studies related to brain aging.

DHA is mainly found in three areas of the body: the brain, the testes, and the retina—all places that have high metabolic activity. We focused specifically on the role of DHA in brain function. In our MAP study, we tracked participants' seafood consumption, followed their cognitive abilities over time, and then analyzed their brains postmortem, looking specifically for neuropathologies and high mercury levels. While we did find higher levels of mercury among those who ate fish, overall seafood consumption (and therefore, higher levels of DHA) was correlated with slower cognitive decline and less Alzheimer's disease pathology.[6] We were very happy to see that there wasn't an increased risk for developing neuropathologies from the mercury levels. So, the evidence comes out strongly in favor of eating fish for the prevention of cognitive decline.

What about fish oil supplements? When it comes to fish oil supplements, the clinical trials have not shown benefits to the brain.

This may be because those studies haven't specifically targeted people who are not fish eaters. This detail is important because non-fish-eaters would have very low levels of omega 3s in their system already. But when testing people who already have adequate levels of omega-3s, you may not see a change in benefits to the brain. More research is needed.

3. Folate

Folate is the B vitamin known as B_9. You've probably heard about this nutrient being crucial during early pregnancy to reduce the risk of birth defects of the brain and spine. Deficiencies in folate have been shown to increase homocysteine levels in the blood, which can cause inflammation. Homocysteine is an amino acid that is broken down by folate and other B vitamins in the body and converted to other nutrients your body needs. Study after study has shown that low blood levels of folate are associated with an increased risk of developing heart disease, stroke, and Alzheimer's disease.[7]

What about folate supplements? If you are very low in this particular nutrient, then taking a supplement to get yourself up to an adequate level is important. Studies on supplements that evaluated people who were either deficient or marginal in folate show a link between reduction of homocysteine levels and improvement in cognitive outcomes with a folate supplement.[8] Always check with your doctor before considering a dietary supplement.

4. Vitamin B_{12}

Vitamin B_{12} plays a crucial role in the brain's normal functioning. One of the symptoms of vitamin B_{12} deficiency syndrome is in fact memory impairment. Vitamin B_{12} is essential to the formation and maintenance of myelin, a fatty sheath that covers the axons of neurons and enhances electrical impulses of neurotransmission. Deficiencies in either folate or vitamin B_{12} increase homocysteine levels, and high levels of homocysteine in the blood can cause inflammation and atherosclerosis—both risk factors for Alzheimer's disease. There are different conditions that can cause deficiencies; however, many more middle-aged and older adults have insufficient levels of vitamin B_{12}. This can be due to less efficient absorption (common with aging), low intake of vitamin B_{12}–containing foods, excessive alcohol consumption, or medications that make absorbing the vitamin more difficult. This vitamin is obtained almost exclusively from animal products, such as meat, fish, eggs, cheese, and milk. Middle-aged adults, older adults, and individuals who follow a vegan diet would do well to have their physicians check whether their levels of vitamin B_{12} are low or low-normal.

5. Unsaturated Fats

There are four major dietary fats in the human diet: saturated fats, trans fats, monounsaturated fats, and polyunsaturated fats. Saturated fat is solid at room temperature. It most often comes from animal products, such as butter, cheese, red meat, and commercially baked goods. Studies indicate that these fats can impair the blood-brain barrier, which is important for keeping harmful free radicals out of the brain as well as for transporting essential nutrients in, while escorting the waste out.

Trans fats can be either naturally occurring or synthetic. Naturally occurring trans fats are produced in the gut of some animals, such as cows, and are in foods made from these animals (like milk and meat products). Artificial trans fats are made from the hydrogenation of vegetable oils. They improve the shelf life of food products and can also improve food texture and flavor. But the downside is that they increase LDL (bad) cholesterol and decrease HDL (good) cholesterol—this is a known risk factor for Alzheimer's disease.

Studies that have investigated the connection between fats and dementia and cognitive decline consistently show that a diet high in saturated fat and trans fat can double or triple the risk of developing Alzheimer's.[9] However, if you have a higher ratio of mono- and polyunsaturated fats to saturated fats, that can decrease your risk.

What we can take from all of this is that the type of fat you consume is important. Reducing or minimizing the amount of saturated fats and trans fats in your diet and increasing the amount of monounsaturated fats (found in olive oil, nuts, olives, and avocados) and polyunsaturated fats (like omega 3s from salmon, albacore tuna, and other fatty fish) is best for brain health.

THE "BENEFICIAL" NUTRIENTS

Other nutrients seem to be promising for protecting cognitive health, but at this point we just have too few studies, or the evidence is inconsistent. Nevertheless, they do carry other health benefits for the body. These nutrients include the following:

1. **Carotenoids**, particularly beta-carotene and lutein, have been linked to dementia prevention.[10] They can be found in abundance in leafy green vegetables as well as yellow, orange, and red fruits and vegetables. As a dietary constituent, carotenoids act as antioxidants, protecting cells from free-radical damage. The almost 600 known types of carotenoids are all fat-soluble, which means your body absorbs their nutrients best when consumed with fat.

2. **Polyphenols** are naturally occurring compounds found in plants. They can alleviate oxidative stress by acting as direct scavengers of free radicals, and can aid in repair of DNA

damage. **Flavonoids**, one class of polyphenols, are a diverse group of phytonutrients (plant chemicals) found in many fruits and vegetables. They have been reported to improve learning and memory by enhancing neuron function, protecting vulnerable neurons, and promoting the formation of new neurons in the brain. They also have beneficial anti-inflammatory effects, protecting cells from the oxidative damage that can lead to disease. Studies have shown that flavonoids may be responsible for reducing neuroinflammation in the brain and that dietary flavonoids may reduce risk for Alzheimer's disease.[11]

3. **Vitamin D** is another fat-soluble vitamin. Vitamin D deficiency has been linked to a host of health conditions, like osteoporosis, diabetes, cancers, and hypertension.[12] In a study from the MAP cohort, researchers found that higher levels of the active form of vitamin D were associated with better cognitive performance prior to death; much more research is needed to understand these relationships.[13] Vitamin D promotes calcium absorption in the gut, so when ingested with calcium, it may help prevent osteoporosis in older adults. Sun exposure is a great way to get vitamin D, and so are a few select foods like fortified milk and orange juice. Some factors, such as obesity, make metabolizing vitamin D more difficult. And those with darker skin, those with liver and kidney impairment, and the elderly have a harder time absorbing vitamin D from the sun's rays.

CHAPTER 3

The MIND Diet and Its Evidence for Protection against Neurodegenerative Diseases

By 2015, the studies on nutrition's relation to brain health had been mostly observational. For example, in the CHAP and MAP studies, we took people in the community and asked them questions about their diet and lifestyle patterns and evaluated them for disease, but we didn't ask them to change anything. We could surmise that when people have high-quality diets, they are more likely to take good care of their health—they go to the doctor, take medications they might need, are more socially active, and exercise more regularly. Yet it was difficult to say whether diet alone was causing or preventing disease. To better understand the link between diet and its effect on brain health, I knew a dietary intervention trial was needed. Since my colleagues and I had gathered a significant amount of evidence through CHAP and MAP, I thought it was the right time for a randomized controlled trial on food's connection to dementia.

In the research world, the randomized controlled trial is considered the "Cadillac" study design. Here scientists randomly assign people to a certain diet. All those commingling factors—exercising, being socially active, going to the doctor, taking medications, and so on—are also accounted for, so that we can be sure our results are directly linked to the diet and not other things.

Before we embarked on our trial, we had to determine the exact diet we'd test with our participants. At that point, the two diets that had been studied the most were the Mediterranean diet and the **D**ietary **A**pproaches to **S**top **H**ypertension (DASH) diet. Both had already been shown to prevent cardiovascular conditions, hypertension, and illnesses such as diabetes, which, as we mentioned earlier, are known risk factors for Alzheimer's. Although each of these diets had also shown benefits in preventing cognitive decline, there did not exist a single dietary pattern that incorporated the foods we found to have the most evidence for protecting the aging brain. My team and I, including Dr. Christy Tangney, along with Dr. Frank Sacks, one of the originators of the DASH diet and a former mentor of mine at the Harvard School of Public Health, decided to bridge this gap in the scientific community.

We took the best of those two popular diets and modified them to reflect the most compelling scientific evidence on the connection between nutrition and the brain. The result: a hybrid between the Mediterranean and DASH diets, the **M**editerranean-DASH **I**ntervention for **N**eurodegenerative **D**elay diet, or the MIND diet.

Before we tested the MIND diet in a randomized controlled trial, we set out to investigate this diet pattern in relation to cognitive aging[1] as well as a diagnosis of Alzheimer's disease[2] in one of our population studies. This would help us gather further evidence, which would better our chances of securing funding for the clinical trial. Remember the MAP study? This is the study where we collected comprehensive dietary assessments on food and nutrient intake, using a food frequency questionnaire, and repeated it on an annual basis. We were able to use these dietary reports to assign a score to rank how well people followed each of the dietary recommendations specified in the MIND diet. We divided foods into 10 brain-healthy groups and 5 brain-unhealthy ones. There were several components for scoring that ranged from 0 (lowest adherence) to 15 (highest adherence). Participants' diets were assessed using the MIND diet score, which was a tally of brain-healthy and brain-unhealthy foods consumed on a weekly basis.

Our analysis was based on 923 participants who at the baseline did not have Alzheimer's disease and who had already provided dietary data, so we could assign a MIND diet score; then we looked for the development of new Alzheimer's cases over the course of 5 years. The participants ranged in age from 58 to 98 years old and had anywhere from two to five assessments to measure cognitive change throughout this time period. During these assessments, neurophysiological technicians administered a battery of 19 cognitive tests, so we had a very detailed measure of how well their brains functioned over time.

The first reports from the MAP study on the MIND diet came out in 2015. The results showed that the participants who were in the top third of MIND diet scores on the scale of 15 (8.5 to 12.5, with 12.5 being the highest score obtained) had a 53 percent lower risk of developing Alzheimer's disease than those with the lowest MIND scores (2.5 to 6.5). Another significant finding was that those who scored in the intermediate range (scores of 7.0 to 8.0) had a 35 percent lower risk of developing Alzheimer's disease. When I saw these results, I was excited to dive deeper into what the MIND diet was doing to protect the brain.

In the second report from the MAP study, we looked at whether the MIND diet score was associated with changes in cognitive abilities over the course of a decade. Participants were assigned a MIND diet score based on their first diet assessments, and then we followed them for up to 10 years to see whether a high or low score could be linked to cognitive decline over time. We found that people who scored in the top third for closely following the MIND diet had very little change in their cognitive abilities over time. They were the equivalent of 7.5 years younger in age compared to people who scored in the lowest range.

In further analysis of the MAP study cohort, we evaluated how the MIND diet compared to the Mediterranean and DASH diets in relation to neuroprotection. We reanalyzed the MAP participants' dietary assessments to calculate scores for how closely they followed the DASH and Mediterranean diets. We then related these scores to our measures of cognitive decline and the development of Alzheimer's. Although both the Mediterranean and DASH diets were associated with slower cognitive decline and a lower risk of developing Alzheimer's disease, the MIND diet was twice as protective of cognitive decline. High scores on the MIND and Mediterranean diets correlated with a more than 50 percent risk reduction in Alzheimer's disease, but even those with moderate scores on the MIND diet had a 35 percent risk reduction. Neither of the other two diets had such a reduction with moderate scores.

There seemed to be a strong association between the MIND diet and reducing Alzheimer's risk, which was really exciting. We devised a diet and it worked in this study. But the results needed to be confirmed by other investigations and through a randomized controlled trial. This was the best way to establish a cause-and-effect relationship between the MIND diet and reductions in the incidence of Alzheimer's disease.

The evidence from this population study helped secure funding from the National Institute on Aging, a division of the National Institutes of Health, for the subsequent trial set to begin in 2016. This study would be a comprehensive investigation to test the ability of the MIND diet to slow cognitive decline and would set the stage for an ongoing investigation to explore risk for Alzheimer's disease and related dementias.[3]

CHAPTER 4

The MIND Diet Intervention to Prevent Alzheimer's Disease

The MIND diet intervention trial was an exciting moment for the world of research in nutrition and Alzheimer's prevention. The results of this trial are important to our understanding of preventive strategies for Alzheimer's, and directions for future research on a relatively new topic of scientific exploration. It was a multiyear collaboration between Rush University Medical Center, Harvard T. H. Chan School of Public Health, and Brigham and Women's Hospital in Boston.

The MIND study team successfully enrolled 604 participants and assigned them to either the group that would follow the MIND diet or the comparator group, where they would follow their usual diet and not alter the types of foods they regularly consumed. Yet participants in both diet groups were encouraged to reduce overall intake by 250 calories per day to promote mild weight loss. It was important for us to coach both groups toward weight loss, so that all participants received valuable health recommendations. Both groups had the same intensity of coaching from their assigned registered dietitians, who guided them to follow one of these two plans, with mild caloric reduction (largely through portion control guidelines), mindful eating strategies, and other behavioral techniques.

The participants ranged in age from 65 to 84, with the average age being 70. They had no cognitive impairment at baseline, although they all had a family history of dementia and had suboptimal diets with a body mass index (BMI) of 25 or greater, putting them in the overweight category. But they were relatively healthy and representative of a general population at risk for Alzheimer's disease. We did not exclude individuals who had hypertension, diabetes, or moderate levels of heart disease, since our purpose was to target modifiable risk factors (lifestyle behaviors within one's control to change) for cognitive decline and development of Alzheimer's. Having high blood pressure, high cholesterol, and obesity (particularly in midlife) increases one's probability of getting dementia later in life. The main aim was to test the hypothesis that the MIND diet slows the decline in cognition. To test this, we administered a large battery of tests that are used to measure cognitive abilities.

The participants of this study were highly motivated—nearing the end of the trial, we had over a 95 percent retention rate (to put this in perspective, most studies strive to retain 80 percent of their participants!). I am humbled by the hard work these participants did for the trial and for the public and am so grateful for their dedication. They realize that so many people, in the United States and all over the world, will benefit from the study's results.

Note from Laura Morris

In late summer of 2019, my mother discovered she had advanced cancer, and was told she had only months left to live. As a world leader on health and disease prevention, and as a person who practiced healthy living over the course of her life, this came as devastating news. Not only was the MIND diet trial nearing completion, she also was a principal investigator or co-investigator of more than a half dozen NIH-funded studies of nutrition and its effects on Alzheimer's disease and other neurological conditions. As we all sat in a state of shock over her diagnosis, she set to work to hand over her life's work to trusted colleagues to carry on the research. Not surprisingly, she did not care to sit in a space of despair; as she said, "There is so much work to be done."

My mother died on February 15, 2020, at the age of 64. Less than one month later, COVID-19 was declared a global pandemic. Immediately following this declaration, the world went into lockdown. Children stayed home from school, all nonessential businesses closed, and people were told not to socialize, hug, or stand within 6 feet of another person outside their household. The news showed daily counts of people who contracted the virus and where clusters of the virus were. Hospitals all over the world were over capacity or ran out of supplies and were unable to treat patients with the virus. Young, healthy people were being put on ventilators in the ICU. Masks and facial coverings were required to be worn everywhere—for some, even outside. The terms "contactless delivery," "social distancing," and "quarantine" became everyday phrases. The effects of all this were devastating to our way of life, our mental functioning, and our ability to maintain our health. Year 1 of this global pandemic marked the beginning of year 3, the final year, of the MIND diet trial.

For my mother, the MIND diet trial was another layer of that onion we peel back to increase our understanding of nutrition and the aging brain. My mother's hope for the MIND diet trial was that we would have new discoveries, along with ways to improve research methods and another step forward in the study of Alzheimer's prevention. My biggest regret is that she doesn't get to see the different layers she loved to peel back to find more questions that need answering, and getting one step closer in our understanding of the role nutrition has on this disease. Mom was the type of person who always looked for the light and love in every situation. In her final days of life she said, "I cannot believe the life I have had. I had a career that I loved and gave me purpose, I had the most wonderful husband and children a person could ask for, I had the most amazing friends. I have had the most magical life."

CHAPTER 5

The Loss of a Great Leader

By Jennifer Ventrelle

In the spring of 2016, I was honored to be invited by Dr. Martha Clare Morris to be the lead dietitian for the MIND diet intervention trial. That meant I was charged with the task of using our knowledge about the potential for whole foods (not drugs!) to make a positive impact in the field of Alzheimer's disease research—and figuring out how to get people to learn about the diet, adopt it, and enjoy it enough to integrate it into their lifestyle for 3 years. We were coaching people in both groups to lose weight, so everybody got something out of this experiment. I felt like I'd been handed a map to a bottomless pot of gold at the end of the rainbow, and I was responsible for leading a select group of older adults straight to it.

To be working with one of the leading experts in the field of nutrition and dementia was a true highlight in my career as a registered dietitian. Dr. Morris invited me to join her team on the first of many trials that she envisioned in her development of the MIND Center for Brain Health at Rush University Medical Center.

For 4 years, I worked very closely with Dr. Morris, watching her show up every day with bright-eyed enthusiasm and a welcoming smile. She would make every decision with sheer passion—from deciding on big issues that would affect the way we conducted our research, to making small decisions like the best color fabric for the new chairs in the waiting room. Next to spending time with her children and grandchildren, this work was truly her happiest place.

The untimely passing of Dr. Morris in February 2020 happened just before all in-person research operations were suspended due to the COVID-19 pandemic shutdown. For all intents and purposes, the whole world as we knew it seemed to be suspended in time. Fear of an unknown future for everyone, from older adults to unborn children, settled in and felt like a heavy weight resting on all our shoulders. To say that this was a traumatic period in history would truly be an understatement.

Although the intervention activities remained remote until the end of the trial, it was important to the integrity of the research design to get back to in-person outcome assessment visits as quickly as safely possible, since it is not possible to perfectly replicate the cognitive measurements with remote methods. In July 2020, the operations team began to prepare for a staggered reentry back into the office, limiting the planned number of assessment visits to three per day and the number of staff in the office to five per day. Some participants understandably refused to come for in-person visits during this time but wanted to remain in the study until they felt comfortable with closer interaction, resulting in additional intervention contacts, delays in final visit assessments far beyond the originally scheduled dates, and the creation of different timelines for some participants compared to the original protocol.

As you can imagine, COVID-19 presented plenty of impediments for keeping a clinical trial on track, but luckily we were able to adapt in the presence of uncertainty. I am proud of everyone on our research team, who managed to guide participants to follow their prescribed plan in the face of a pandemic and come into the office to complete in-person assessments, all while worrying about their own health and safety within a few short months of losing our leader.

The results of the MIND diet trial were published in the *New England Journal of Medicine* in the summer of 2023.[1] The results showed that by the end of the 3-year trial period, both the MIND diet group and the usual diet group *improved* their cognitive scores on average, as opposed to experiencing cognitive decline. It's remarkable that average scores in both diet groups showed improvement in cognition, since we were expecting to see decline. Although some of the increases in scores may be due to what's called "practice effects," meaning participants may have gotten better at answering the questions in the cognitive battery, we could at least conclude that cognition did not decline over the 3 years. However, this left everyone wondering why there wasn't a big difference seen based on the diets followed.

The beginning of year 3 marked the first year of the global pandemic, a time when following any type of healthy lifestyle guidelines became incredibly challenging for all of us, so we were pleasantly surprised to find that adherence to the weight loss protocol was confirmed in both groups as planned. The average weight loss in both groups reached 5.5 percent at 6 months (exceeding the 3 to 5 percent target), and participants in both groups were able to maintain this loss through the end of the 3-year intervention, even in the face of the pandemic. The original plan was for the MIND group to work toward weight loss while following the MIND diet and for the control group to work toward weight loss without changing the type of foods they ate. We learned, however, that both groups improved their diets. The MIND group's average score increased to 11.1, and even the control group's average score increased to 8.5. The increase in MIND score as representative of a brain-healthy diet was confirmed in both groups with measurements of blood biomarkers showing average increases in alpha and beta-carotene, lutein, and zeaxanthin. This score of 8.5 for the control group was important. According to the MAP studies, this number equates to a 53 percent reduced risk for Alzheimer's disease[2] and is associated with the cognitive functioning equivalent of individuals 7.5 years younger.[3] This suggests that the control group reached a "therapeutic" MIND score that may have positively influenced their cognition by the end of the trial.

Although the average score in the MIND group was still higher compared to the control, it did not turn out to be a statistically significant difference. From a clinical perspective, it is good news indeed that, like the previous observational research, these results suggest that a MIND score as low as 8.5 may be capable of positively impacting cognition. Of course, more research is needed to confirm this. It is also possible that a time period of greater than 3 years is required in order to detect significant changes in cognition. Earlier research on the MIND diet studied people for up to 10 years to detect these brain changes.

It is important to note that it is very difficult to design dietary intervention studies with an appropriate control group. In a clinical trial, the purpose of a control group is to be able to describe any changes that happen in the treatment group as a result of the treatment, rather than as a result of any other circumstances. For example, in a drug trial, one group would take the active drug, while the other group would take a placebo pill. Participants and researchers agree to be "blinded" to which individuals are taking the active drug and which are taking the placebo so as not to influence the outcome of the trial—intentionally or unintentionally. It is not nearly as simple to do this in a diet intervention trial, since researchers and participants must know what types of foods to prescribe and eat.

In addition, no one could have predicted the impact of the effects of COVID-19. It's possible that the temporary disruption of study operations during the lockdown—including required modifications to the study protocol, outcomes testing, and overall pandemic-related stressors on the participants and study staff—could have impacted the results of the trial. Future research will explore the role of the MIND diet compared to a more typical control, similar to a usual care setting such as doctor's office visits, other healthcare providers that do not offer as much support as was received in the trial, or a less intensive self-guided program, in the absence of a global pandemic.

I often imagine what Dr. Morris would make of the results of a 3-year trial that were complicated by the effects of COVID-19. We can't ever know for sure, but I suspect she would simply consider it another layer of the onion peeled back, propelling her forward to further explore the role of diet and cognitive functioning for the sake of the research team, the participants in the MIND trial, and the entire field of nutrition and dementia. Good scientists conduct research with complete equipoise, aware of the possibility that the final outcome of a study may not perfectly align with the original hypothesis due to any number of circumstances. Great scientists see the success in *all* outcomes as an opportunity for future explorations and a contribution to public health. I feel lucky to have worked under the leadership of a great scientist.

CHAPTER 6

Exciting New Research
on the MIND Diet

By Jennifer Ventrelle

Many studies have taken the initiative to explore a wider lifestyle approach on the outcome of cognitive decline and dementia. According to a report in the *Lancet*, one of the world's most reputable scientific journals, an updated cluster of modifiable risk factors, based on the most recent research in the field, has the potential to prevent or delay up to 40 percent of dementias.[1]

The first study to explore a multidomain lifestyle approach occurred prior to the MIND trial. The Finnish Geriatric Intervention Study to Prevent Cognitive Impairment and Disability (FINGER) study explored diet, physical activity, cognitive training, and cardiovascular risk factor management and showed positive results on cognitive functioning in older adults at risk for dementia.[2] FINGER set the groundwork for the U.S. Study to Protect Brain Health through Lifestyle Intervention to Reduce Risk (U.S. POINTER). Like all great researchers, Dr. Morris had already begun exploring these additional factors in the midst of the MIND trial. She linked up with Dr. Laura Baker at Wake Forest University School of Medicine, who launched the five-site randomized controlled trial in the fall of 2018 to explore an "Americanized" version of the FINGER trial using the MIND diet

RISK FACTORS FOR ALZHEIMER'S DISEASE	
Nonmodifiable	**Modifiable**
Older age	Overweight/obesity
APOE-ε4 genotype	High blood pressure
Head injury	High cholesterol
	Diabetes
	Unhealthy diet
	Physical inactivity
	Low engagement in cognitive and social activities
	Depression
	Less education
	Hearing impairment
	Smoking
	Excessive alcohol consumption
	Head injury
	Air pollution

as part of the dietary intervention component of the multidomain lifestyle intervention. With the U.S. POINTER study, the United States is one of more than 30 countries involved in World-Wide FINGERS, the first worldwide initiative for prevention of Alzheimer's disease and related dementias, which is led by Dr. Miia Kivipelto.[3]

The U.S. POINTER study is a continued exploration of the MIND diet, with the added lifestyle factors of physical activity, cognitive and social engagement, and self-monitoring of health metrics. I'm thrilled to be a part of the team, codirecting the interventions for all five US sites. Now, with the help of leaders like Dr. Baker and Dr. Christy Tangney, one of the original creators of the MIND diet, we can carry on Dr. Morris's vision to test the effects of diet among other lifestyle factors in diverse communities across the United States and throughout the world.

Dr. Tangney and Dr. Neelum Aggarwal at Rush University Medical Center are the first to lead a clinical trial to explore the MIND diet in stroke survivors. The basis for this trial was built again by looking at data from the MAP study, this time examining individuals who had a history of stroke.[4] It was found that those who achieved a MIND diet score between 9.0 and 10.5 had a slower rate of cognitive decline after a stroke. The current clinical trial will determine whether the MIND diet can offer a direct and clinically significant additive benefit to usual post-stroke care.

I'm grateful to have the opportunity to help carry on Dr. Morris's vision of future explorations with the existing team of researchers in the ongoing trials mentioned above and humbled to be her co-author on this book.

WHY CHOOSE THE MIND DIET?

Research suggests that the MIND diet may be an even more effective way to protect the brain from cognitive decline than either the Mediterranean or DASH diets alone.[5] A wide body of research also points to Mediterranean-type diets as the best strategy for long-term weight loss.[6] For patients who are overweight or obese, doctors have been encouraged to begin by prescribing Mediterranean-DASH type diets before turning to medications, weight loss surgeries, or very-low-calorie diets.[7] The MIND diet is a Mediterranean-DASH dietary pattern that has been shown to be associated with a slowed rate of cognitive decline and delayed onset of Alzheimer's disease. So, when the preliminary research on the diet was published and Dr. Morris received her grant from the National Institute on Aging to conduct the MIND trial—the first ever clinical trial to explore the direct relationship between diet and cognitive decline—everyone was thrilled.

When Dr. Morris received the grant, she was encouraged to copyright "the MIND diet" so that the information would remain confidential until the results of the trial were officially published. This would also mean that other institutions would have to pay a fee to access the diet. But Dr. Morris was a true public health advocate. She thought that science should be accessible to everyone and did not heed this advice. Unfortunately, that meant that anyone could pub-lish inaccurate or incomplete information and call it "the MIND diet." In fact, if you do a quick Google search now, you'll find more than half a dozen books *other than* those written by Dr. Morris. We urge you to be selective in all the health information you consume and consider the source, including diet books. The diet industry is one of the most notoriously polluted for misinformation. For infor-mation regarding the development and initial findings on the MIND diet, Dr. Morris and her team are the most qualified to deliver the facts and will be the best guides to help you implement and get the most out of the diet. Dr. Morris's first book, *Diet for the MIND,* was based on the initial background research leading up to the MIND diet intervention trial.

Although the results of the first clinical trial suggest that even more research is needed, we can see that following the MIND diet at a moderate level coupled with weight loss efforts and a strong support partner for 3 years can have positive effects on brain health and may actually help improve cognition. Other researchers continue to work with the MAP study data to better understand the diet's potential impact on cognitive decline and the more long-term outcome of Alzheimer's disease.

Dr. Thomas Holland, an assistant professor at Rush University Medical Center, worked with researchers to explore participants' intake of flavonols (a class of flavonoid polyphenols with powerful antioxidant effects) from leafy green vegetables, some other vegeta-bles such as broccoli, and berries. Higher intakes of bioactives (com-pounds found in plants that can be health promoting) contained in these foods were associated with slower rates of cognitive decline.[8]

Dr. Puja Agarwal, a nutritional epidemiologist at Rush University Medical Center, took an even closer look by exploring the pathology of brain tissue of the participants from the MAP study who donated their brains after death. This approach allows for more direct insight into the link between diet and risk for Alzheimer's disease. In this analysis, it was discovered that both the MIND and Mediterranean diets were associated with fewer signs of Alzheimer's disease pathology—most notably, beta-amyloid load, thought to be the hallmark of Alzheimer's disease.[9] Specific patterns that stood out were the power of the MIND diet's leafy green vegetables and their association with lower levels of plaques versus the higher levels found in brain tissue of individuals who ate high amounts of fried foods and sweets and pastries. Those who followed the MIND diet most closely compared to the lowest level had average amyloid plaques similar to individuals 12 years younger. Dr. Agarwal took the same approach with this population once again and found that the brain tissue of those who had the highest intake of a bioactive component called pelargonidin, found in strawberries, was associated with the fewest phosphorylated tau tangles, another Alzheimer's disease pathology marker.[10] As great researchers never stop exploring and searching for new answers, more evidence continues to surface on the potential benefits of this dietary pattern.

The MIND diet recommends foods to eat and foods to limit based on the most rigorously investigated research to protect the brain from disease. In addition, these foods may help prevent heart disease, diabetes, obesity, and other chronic conditions that increase the risk of Alzheimer's disease. Following this diet is simple and adaptable to almost any lifestyle. The MIND diet continues to rank on *U.S. News & World Report*'s Best Diets list. In 2023, it was ranked #3 for best plant-based diet and #4 in best family-friendly diet and best diet overall.[11]

In this book, we will introduce you to nutritious disease-fighting foods and tell you where to find them, how to prepare them, and how often to consume them. Once you have a good understanding of the foods to eat and the foods to limit, you will learn essential tools to help incorporate these foods into your weekly routine. Next, we will highlight the most effective practices for keeping you accountable, finding support, and taking steps toward losing weight. Most importantly, we will show you how to plan effectively so you can manage all that life throws at you while maintaining your health and nutrition needs. With all of this acquired knowledge and these practical tips, you will be ready to start the Official MIND Diet 6-Week Program. The program is designed to help you take small, sustainable steps toward incorporating the foods to eat and reducing the foods to limit. With the most up-to-date scientific methods for brain protection and weight loss, our intention for you is that by the end of this program you'll be armed with knowledge on the most nutritious foods, have access to more than 60 tasty and easy-to-prepare recipes, and be able to create a personalized plan that will easily integrate the MIND diet into your current lifestyle to aid you on your journey toward optimal health and well-being.

PART II

FOODS FOR BRAIN HEALTH

By Jennifer Ventrelle

"Your brain uses nutrients to form the cell's individual parts, to provide the fuel and build the proteins that it needs to function, and to protect the brain's neurons against injury—and we acquire these nutrients from foods we eat."

—*Dr. Martha Clare Morris*

CHAPTER 7

NeverMIND the Diet

"The MIND diet has been more helpful than WeightWatchers as I feel there is a purpose for following the diet. Weight-Watchers has been a long and boring approach to losing weight, as I never got into doing the program. Sometimes I would just count the points mindlessly, and then feel bad if I ate the wrong things. Now, with the MIND diet, I know what is good and what isn't, and then move on if I've eaten the wrong foods."

—*Faye M.*

I had an opportunity to witness the difficulty in changing lifestyle behaviors firsthand. My mother, who grew up in Italy, would make home-cooked meals every night and show her boundless love for us through huge portions of homemade lasagna, fried meatballs, and freshly baked chocolate chip cookies. Unfortunately, I saw my father enjoy those deliciously heavy meals with a cigarette as both an appetizer and a dessert. The man smoked roughly five packs of cigarettes a day and, over the course of his short 45 years on this earth, endured a series of seven heart attacks, a triple bypass surgery, and a heart transplant. When he received the new heart, he rationalized that he may be healthy enough to take up smoking again, but it turns out the rest of his body wasn't so resilient.

At age 13, I committed to having some sort of career where I could help save people like my father from an early death.

I went on to become a registered dietitian and earned a master's degree from a competitive research-based accredited dietetics program at Rush University, the same institution where Dr. Morris began her career and created the MIND diet. I was an idealist and assumed that, with my extensive training, I'd be able to educate people to make significant health improvements. But it turns out the old adage "knowledge is power" isn't really true unless people are motivated to apply that knowledge and the support to keep going. It was a tough lesson to learn. During my first job at Rush's outpatient clinic, I would take it personally when, after I spent time talking to people about their high cholesterol or diabetes, outlining clear steps to manage their conditions, they usually came back without following through on their goals. Many didn't return at all.

After I got some experience under my belt and was able to better listen to my clients, I noticed that people often love the novelty of a new diet or program. They get excited while embarking on a plan, but then feel discouraged when life gets in the way and they're unable to "stick to the plan." They feel like they've failed, and that doesn't feel good. Not many of us continue to do things that don't feel good...at least not for very long.

After about 10 years working with other dietitians, I was fortunate enough to expand my role to a more multidisciplinary team with researchers, physicians, and behavioral psychologists. I feel grateful for this time, as it helped me understand that the assumption that one diet is optimal for everyone ignores the reality that people are influenced by food preferences, cultural or religious traditions, food availability, and food intolerances. We have a lot of research supporting this as well.[1] In other words, it's easy to sit in the doctor's (or dietitian's) office and say that you're going to follow a diet. But when the plan doesn't allow chocolate cake on your birthday or fails to recognize how much you love your mom's homemade spaghetti (despite the carb count), or causes you to shell out twice as much at the grocery

48

store, it makes it pretty tough to commit to a "lifestyle" defined by the plan.

Eventually I realized that my job isn't to "save" anybody. We all have a personal responsibility to care for ourselves, as long as we are of sound mind and body, in the best way we know how. And hopefully we can give ourselves a little compassion and let up on the pressure to be perfect. In my practice today, I strive to release all judgment, meet people wherever they are, educate them to the best of my professional ability, and empower them to make their own choices. My intention in this book is to give you reliable, scientifically sound information as it relates to nutrition, cognition, and weight management with practical recommendations for an eating pattern that I find fits into "real life." To do this, I've teamed up with Laura Morris to create a 6-week program that contains all the tools you'll need to make the MIND diet work for you, along with more than 50 recipes crafted in Laura's very own kitchen. Your job is to choose which (if any) of the suggestions you'd like to implement. My hope is that those of you who do feel ready and inspired to give the MIND diet a try will incorporate it into your life easily, without feeling restricted from your favorite foods, guilty when indulgences happen, and demotivated after the novelty wears off.

The best place to start is with your own mind—that is, your perspective. I've been helping people lose weight and improve eating behaviors for over 20 years, and among the most successful were those who had what I call a *"nondiet"* approach. This is where success is defined as generally keeping to an eating pattern while changing a few key lifestyle habits, versus committing to a strict set of rules that forces you to count calories, eliminate whole food groups, or restrict eating to an arbitrary window of time while using preportioned color-coded containers or some other elaborate system. Instead, the MIND diet recommendations are meant to be specific enough to stay true to their research-based foundation but also broad enough to allow you to fit them into an existing lifestyle. In other words, even though we refer to this eating pattern as the MIND "diet," NeverMIND the Diet!

"When I started the program, I was retired. As you get older, you think you've lost the opportunity to learn about yourself.... The MIND diet brought purpose into my life again. I'd like to thank the founders...not only for older people, but for younger people...to give them a chance at a longer and healthier life.... It's not only changed my life, but the lives of those around me as well."

—*Qamar M.*

THE MIND DIET QUIZ: IS YOUR DIET PROTECTING YOU FROM ALZHEIMER'S DISEASE?

To start to become familiar with the MIND diet foods, complete the quiz below based on your typical intake of food over the past year.

- Beginning in the far left column, notice the food item category, examples that fall within each category, and the serving size of each item. For example, strawberries are included in the list of "berries," and 1 serving is equivalent to ½ cup.

- Use the second column to determine how often you eat each food item on a weekly basis. You may eat some foods more regularly at certain times of the year compared to others. Just try to answer the question based on the average across the whole year. For example, if you eat ½ cup of berries 4 times per week, but only when they're in season, you might consider your intake to be closer to 1 or 2 servings per week on average for the whole year.

- The third column will determine the points you've earned for each individual food item. For example, if you eat 1 to 4 servings of berries per week, you've earned 0.5 points for this food item.

- Write the number of points you've earned for each food item in the fourth column, labeled "Your Food Points."

- Add up all the numbers in the fourth column to get your MIND diet score.

- Check the "Research Shows" box on page 54 to see if you're getting a "therapeutic" MIND diet score and eating a brain-healthy diet.

Food Items	How often do you eat these foods each week?	Possible Points	Your Food Points
Extra-Virgin Olive Oil (oil used in salad dressing, sautéing or other cooking, etc.) **1 serving = 1 tablespoon**	0–6 servings/week	0	
	7–13 servings/week	0.5	
	14+ servings/week	1	
Fried Foods (potato chips, tortilla chips, french fries, fried chicken, any deep-fried foods, etc.) **1 serving = 1 serving**	0–1 serving/week	1	
	2–3 servings/week	0.5	
	4+ servings/week	0	
Leafy Green Vegetables (spinach, kale, greens, romaine lettuce, etc. — *not* iceberg lettuce) **1 serving = 1 cup raw or ½ cup cooked**	0–2 servings/week	0	
	3–6 servings/week	0.5	
	7+ servings/week	1	
Sweets, Pastries & Sweet Drinks (brownies, candy bars, ice cream, Danishes, doughnuts, cakes, pies, scones, non-diet sodas, juice drinks, sweet tea, coffee drinks, energy drinks, etc.) **1 serving = 1 treat or 8-ounce drink**	0–4 servings/week	1	
	5–6 servings/week	0.5	
	7+ servings/week	0	

Vegetables Other than Leafy Greens (broccoli, carrots, onions, peppers, green beans, tomatoes, yams, squash, beets, etc. — *not* white potatoes) **1 serving = ½ cup, cooked or raw**	0–4 servings/week	0
	5–6 servings/week	0.5
	7+ servings/week	1
Berries (strawberries, blueberries, blackberries, raspberries) **1 serving = ½ cup**	0 servings/week	0
	1–4 servings/week	0.5
	5+ servings/week	1
Fish & Seafood (fish and shellfish such as salmon, tuna, tilapia, cod, halibut, shrimp, crab, lobster, etc. — *not* fried) **1 serving = 3–5 ounces**	0 servings/week	0
	1+ servings/week	1
Poultry (white-meat chicken and turkey — *not* fried) **1 serving = 3–5 ounces without skin/bones**	0 servings/week	0
	1 serving/week	0.5
	2+ servings/week	1
Full-Fat Cheese (cheese on pizza and sandwiches, cream cheese, ricotta, cottage, Parmesan, mozzarella, cheddar, string, etc.) **1 serving = 1 ounce**	0–2 servings/week	1
	3–6 servings/week	0.5
	7+ servings/week	0
Beans & Legumes (black, pinto, kidney, lima, and navy beans; chickpeas; lentils; tofu, edamame, hummus, etc.) **1 serving = ½ cup canned or cooked**	0 servings/week	0
	1–2 servings/week	0.5
	3+ servings/week	1

Nuts & Seeds (almonds, walnuts, cashews, peanuts, pistachios, nut butter, seeds) **1 serving = 1 ounce nuts or seeds or 2 tablespoons nut/seed butter**	0 servings/week	0	
	1–4 servings/week	0.5	
	5+ servings/week	1	
Red Meat & Processed Meat (steak, hamburger, pork, ham, lamb, hot dog, sausage, bacon, bologna, salami, pepperoni, etc.) **1 serving = 3–5 ounces**	0–3 servings/week	1	
	4–6 servings/week	0.5	
	7+ servings/week	0	
Whole Grains (whole-grain bread, pasta, cereal, and crackers; brown rice; quinoa; barley; bulgur; farro; oats; etc.) **1 serving = ½ cup cooked grains or 1 slice bread**	0–4 servings/week	0	
	5–20 servings/week	0.5	
	21+ servings/week	1	
Butter & Stick Margarine (added to bread or vegetables, used in sautéing or other cooking, etc.) **1 serving = 1 teaspoon**	0–7 servings/week	1	
	8–13 servings/week	0.5	
	14+ servings/week	0	
Wine (red wine, white wine, sparkling wine, dessert wine, etc.) **1 serving = 5 fluid ounces**	0 servings/week	0	
	1–6 servings/week	0.5	
	7 servings/week	1	
	8+ servings/week	0	
		YOUR MIND DIET SCORE:	

INTERPRETING YOUR SCORE

If you scored between 13 and 15 on the MIND Diet Quiz, congratulations! This is the highest possible range and what is thought to be the most protective against Alzheimer's disease. Research participants in the early MAP cohort studies did not score this high on average; however, there appears to be a direct linear association between MIND score and reduced risk for Alzheimer's disease. This means that higher MIND diet scores corresponded to lower predicted risk, so we recommend aiming for a score between 13 and 15 for what may be the most protective for prevention of cognitive decline and reduced risk for Alzheimer's disease.[2] If you score between 8.5 and 12.5, this puts you at the level that MAP participants reached, and what has been scientifically shown (so far) to be associated with the greatest reduction in risk—53 percent. A score between 7 and 8 would align your eating patterns with a 35 percent reduced risk for Alzheimer's disease and is still considered a "therapeutic" MIND diet score. You can consider this idea of a "therapeutic" score to mean that your score falls within the range that was considered to be brain healthy. In the MIND trial, the average score for all participants fell between 8.5 and 11.1, which corresponded to an improvement in cognition.[3]

If your score is 6.5 or lower, your eating patterns are not aligned with those shown to reduce risk for Alzheimer's disease. This means that there is room for improvement! Keep this initial score handy so that when you begin following the program, you can see how your risk level improves over time.

Here is a summary of the MIND score ranges and the risk reductions:

RESEARCH SHOWS:

People who had a MIND Diet Score of ...	0–6.5	**7.0–8.0**	**8.5–12.5**	13–15
had a reduced risk for developing Alzheimer's disease by ...	No Reduced Risk	**35% Reduced Risk**	**53% Reduced Risk**	Potentially Greatest Reduced Risk*

*Assumed based on linear association between MIND scores and cognitive outcomes.

Before we jump into the foods exclusive to the MIND diet, I'd like to acknowledge that some classically healthy foods aren't included. This is because our focus is on what the research tells us about a food's direct effect on brain health. You may remember from part I, Dr. Morris described her commitment to recommending only the most "rigorously studied" foods based on the "strongest scientific evidence available." For example, you will not find dairy products on the list of MIND diet *"Foods to Choose,"* because there hasn't been a proven link to dairy and its effect on the brain. Milk and yogurt were not shown to be positively or negatively associated with cognition in the CHAP and MAP studies. Therefore, the MIND team did not see these food items as having enough evidence to be included on the diet. This is also true for eggs, fruits other than berries, avocados, dark chocolate, and unsweetened tea.

But just because a particular food is not officially included, that doesn't mean you shouldn't eat it. As I mentioned before, try not to buy into this notion of looking at foods as either "allowed" or "forbidden." Just do your best to include the 10 *Foods to Choose* in your weekly food choices and consume only in moderation the 5 *Foods to Limit*. A perk of the MIND diet is that no foods are really "off limits." See the list of foods in each category in the following tables.

MIND Diet: 10 Foods to Choose		
Food	Goal Quantities & Serving Sizes	Example & Tips
Leafy Green Vegetables (LG)	1 serving/day 1 serving = 1 cup raw or ½ cup cooked	**Count as LG:** dark leafy greens such as spinach, kale, collards, Swiss chard, mustard greens, turnip greens, dandelion greens, arugula, endive, grape leaves, romaine lettuce, spring mix/mixed greens, bok choy, etc. **Do not count as LG:** iceberg lettuce
Other Vegetables (OV)	1 serving/day 1 serving = ½ cup, cooked or raw	**Count as OV:** asparagus, broccoli, brussels sprouts, cabbage, carrots, cauliflower, celery, eggplant, green beans, iceberg lettuce, Bibb lettuce, mushrooms, onions, okra, pumpkin, snow peas, squash, bell peppers, sweet potatoes, tomatoes/tomato sauce, yams, etc. **Do not count as OV:** white potatoes, vegetable juice

FOODS FOR BRAIN HEALTH

Berries (Ber)	5 servings/week 1 serving = ½ cup	**Count as Ber:** blueberries, strawberries, raspberries, blackberries **Do not count as Ber:** dried berries, cranberry sauce
Extra-Virgin Olive Oil (EVOO)	2 servings/day 1 serving = 1 tablespoon	**Count as EVOO:** oil used in dressings or for sautéing or other cooking **Do not count as EVOO:** olive oil cooking spray, oil blends, butter–olive oil blends, non-extra-virgin olive oil **Tip:** Look for the certification seal (see page 79).
Nuts & Seeds (Nut)	5 servings/week 1 serving = 1 ounce nuts or seeds or 2 tablespoons nut/ seed butter	**Count as Nut:** almonds, walnuts, cashews, peanuts, pistachios, and nut butters; seeds such as pumpkin, chia, flax, sunflower, hemp; and seed butters such as sunflower **Do not count as Nut:** nut milks or nut yogurts, candied nuts, powdered peanut butter **Tip:** Although peanuts are technically legumes, they are included in the nut category due to their nutrient profile.
Fish & Seafood (Fsh)	1 serving/week 1 serving = 3–5 ounces	**Count as Fsh:** salmon, tuna, tilapia, cod, mahi-mahi, halibut, scallops, clams, oysters, shrimp, lobster, etc. **Do not count as Fsh:** fried fish and shellfish **Tip:** Fish with the highest concentration of omega-3 fatty acids include salmon, albacore tuna, sardines, anchovies, and mackerel.
Poultry (Poul)	2 servings/week 1 serving = 3–5 ounces without skin/bones	**Count as Poul:** skinless white-meat chicken or turkey, deli-style chicken or turkey, ground white-meat chicken or turkey **Do not count as Poul:** fried poultry, dark meat, duck (light or dark meat), poultry skin
Whole Grains (WG)	3 servings/day 1 serving = 1 slice bread or ½ cup cooked grains	**Count as WG:** whole-grain breads such as whole wheat and dark rye, brown or wild rice, whole-grain pasta, quinoa, barley, bulgur, farro, oats, whole-grain cereal, whole-grain crackers, popcorn, corn tortillas **Do not count as WG:** "enriched" wheat products **Tip:** Look for the word "whole" to be first on the list of ingredients.

Beans & Legumes (Bn)	3 servings/week 1 serving = ½ cup canned or cooked	**Count as Bn:** black, pinto, cannellini, kidney, lima, red/white, and navy beans; chickpeas; lentils; split peas; tofu, edamame, tempeh, and hummus **Do not count as Bn:** soy yogurt, processed soy-based meat substitutes
Wine (Win)	1 serving/day 1 serving = 5 fluid ounces	**Count as Win:** red wine, white wine, sparkling wine **Do not count as Win:** dessert wine **Tip:** Limit total alcohol consumption to no more than 1 drink/day for women and no more than 2 drinks/day for men. Note that it is **not** recommended to begin drinking wine regularly if you do not currently consume alcohol.

MIND Diet: 5 Foods to Limit

Food	Goal Quantities & Serving Sizes	Example & Tips
Red Meat & Processed Meat (RM)	0–3 servings/week 1 serving = 3–5 ounces	**Count as RM:** beef, roast beef, steak, hamburger, pork, pork belly, ham, lamb, hot dogs, sausages, bacon, bologna, salami, pepperoni, Canadian bacon **Do not count as RM:** pork loin/tenderloin, processed meat alternatives
Butter & Stick Margarine (But)	0–1 serving/day 1 serving = 1 teaspoon	**Count as But:** salted and unsalted butter, margarine sticks, butter–olive oil blends **Do not count as But:** "heart-healthy" buttery spreads in a tub such as Smart Balance, Earth Balance, I Can't Believe It's Not Butter, Benecol **Tip:** Replace butter with EVOO whenever possible.
Full-Fat Cheese (Chs)	0–2 servings/week 1 serving = 1 ounce	**Count as Chs:** full-fat mozzarella, Parmesan, cheddar, Colby, ricotta, cottage, cream cheese, and all other whole-milk cheeses **Do not count as Chs:** low-fat or fat-free cheeses **Tip:** Try cheese substitutes, such as nutritional yeast.

Fried Foods (Fri)	0–1 serving/week	**Count as Fri:** any deep-fried food such as potato chips, tortilla chips, french fries, fried chicken or other fried meat, falafel, hushpuppies, empanadas, etc. **Do not count as Fri:** pan-fried, sautéed, or air-fried foods **Tip:** Invest in an air-fryer if possible.
Sweets, Pastries & Sweet Drinks (Swt)	0–4 servings/week 1 serving = 1 treat or 8-ounce drink	**Count as Swt:** biscuits, cakes, sweet rolls, pies, doughnuts, cookies, brownies, candy bars, ice cream, pudding, milkshakes, and sugar-sweetened beverages such as regular sodas, sports drinks, energy drinks, sweetened waters, coffees, and teas. **Do not count as Swt:** hard candy, gelatin **Tip:** Try frozen berries for dessert.

CALORIES AND THE MACRONUTRIENTS

At the most basic level, the energy provided to the body from food is measured in units called calories. Calories are generated from three different sources—fats, proteins, and carbohydrates—together known as macronutrients. Most people may not think of food in terms of how I will be describing it in the next four chapters—vegetables and fruit (chapter 8), unsaturated fats (chapter 9), proteins (chapter 10), and carbohydrates (chapter 11). Instead, it may feel more natural to think of food the way Laura has outlined the recipes in part V—breakfast (chapter 20), main meals (chapter 21), sides, salads, and snacks (chapter 22), and sweets (chapter 23). I am going to invite you to "retrain your brain" to think about food in a new way or at least to consider the added component of a food "category" within your breakfasts, main meals, and snacks.

A big benefit of thinking about foods in these categories and understanding the nutrients they provide is that it allows you to be intentional with the function you'd like the food to perform in your body. For example, the normal process of digestion occurs when food gets consumed, broken down into nutrients by digestive enzymes, and absorbed into the bloodstream. This process triggers a cascade of nervous system and hormonal signals to convert nutrients to usable energy so that the body can perform daily functions like writing an email or embracing a loved one, and biological functions like allowing the heart to deliver oxygen and nutrients to the brain.

We now know from research how to incorporate key foods and limit others to optimize brain and heart health. We also know how often to eat them, and how to effectively combine them to achieve and maintain a healthy weight. By the time you reach the 6-week program in part IV, you'll be fully prepared with this information, along with other tips and tricks to customize the program to best fit your own lifestyle. So, let's dive in with a look at our food categories—beginning with the most important first!

CHAPTER 8

Vegetables (Plural) and Fruit (Singular)

In the MIND diet there are two different categories for vegetables, while there is just one kind of fruit that has been proven to combat cognitive decline. These categories are leafy green vegetables (LG), other vegetables (OV), and berries (Ber).

Vegetables and Fruit	MIND Food Points	
Leafy Green Vegetables (LG) **Goal:** 1 serving/day **Serving size:** 1 cup raw or ½ cup cooked	0–2 servings/week	0
	3–6 servings/week	0.5
	7+ servings/week	1
Other Vegetables (OV) **Goal:** 1 serving/day **Serving size:** ½ cup, cooked or raw	0–4 servings/week	0
	5–6 servings/week	0.5
	7+ servings/week	1
Berries (Ber) **Goal:** 5 servings/week **Serving size:** ½ cup	0 servings/week	0
	1–4 servings/week	0.5
	5+ servings/week	1

These foods tend to fall by the wayside in the typical American diet. But for the MIND diet, vegetables are so important that we put them in two separate categories. We recommend including them in almost every meal if you can.

Vegetables help the body function at its optimal capacity by help-ing regulate a multitude of biological processes and providing the essential vitamins, minerals, antioxidants, and phytochemicals necessary for the body to survive and the brain to thrive. Vegetables are also very low in calories and fill you up quickly, so they are especially beneficial for those seeking weight loss. In terms of the three macronutrients, vegetables contain a small amount of carbohydrates, an even smaller amount of protein, and virtually no fat.

LEAFY GREEN VEGETABLES

By far, the most powerful food group to protect the brain is leafy green vegetables. Research has found that the benefit for cognitive reserve happens with at least 1 serving per day of green leafy vegetables. What is in leafy greens that make them so healthy? Turns out they are one of the most potent sources of a whole handful of nutrients that are protective for the brain.

MIND DIET TARGET

Go for the Greens

Aim for 1 serving of leafy green vegetables daily.

1 serving = 1 cup raw or ½ cup cooked

Examples: spinach; kale; Swiss chard; collard, dandelion, mustard, turnip, and beet greens; arugula; bok choy; endive; grape leaves; romaine lettuce

---

Leafy greens are packed with carotenoids such as beta-carotene, lutein, flavonoids, and other bioactives that protect vulnerable brain cells against oxidative injury and inflammation and contain folate, a powerful B vitamin that builds DNA and fresh new cells. Leafy greens are also a key ingredient for weight loss since they are high in fiber and take up a lot of space in the stomach. Fiber, along with the physical weight and volume of food in the stomach, creates the physical feeling of fullness and triggers the release of a key satiety hormone, leptin. Leptin sends the chemical message to the brain to alert the body that it's time to stop eating. Leafy greens are also very low-calorie, about 25 calories per cup, making them an excellent MIND food to load up on if weight loss is a goal for you. In the MAP study, people who consumed leafy greens at least six times per week had the cognitive functioning of people 11 years younger.[1] Leafy greens were also found to be the strongest component of the MIND diet associated with the lowest level of beta-amyloid plaques and tau tangles in the brain, those markers previously described as the hallmarks of Alzheimer's disease.[2] Think of leafy greens as the foundation from which to build the rest of your new MINDful eating routine.

As we dive deeper into each food on the diet, I'll give you simple tips on how you can incorporate that food *In a Routine* to help form a habit, as well as ideas for getting the food *In a Rush* for times when planning ahead may not be possible. Then, in part III, we will introduce a method for meal planning, highlighting how easy it can be to follow a brain-healthy diet. Let's get started.

WEIGHT LOSS ON THE MIND?

Fill up on leafy green vegetables to create a physical feeling of fullness and send the chemical message to your brain to let your body know the right time to stop eating.

Leafy greens contain only 25 calories per cup.

HOW TO ENJOY LEAFY GREEN VEGETABLES

In a Routine

Start each dinner or lunch with a leafy green salad. A side salad can be a nice complement to just about any cuisine, or you might try having salad as your main course.

Throughout this book, we will be giving you a ton of formal "recipes" (stay tuned for part V!); however, you don't need to follow a formal recipe to incorporate the MIND foods on a routine basis. Here are some "assembled recipe" routines you might try:

- **Revamp Taco Tuesday.** Load up all your fixings (onions, peppers, lean ground taco meat, low-fat shredded cheese, olives, salsa, and guacamole) onto a bed of shredded romaine or red leaf lettuce instead of taco shells.

- **Try lettuce wraps.** Roll low-fat Swiss cheese and turkey with avocado, tomato, and hummus inside a romaine lettuce leaf for a satisfying wrap without sacrificing your waistline.

- **Go stir-fry.** Use collard greens or bok choy instead of rice or noodles as a base, then add veggies, any protein (chicken, shrimp, lean beef, etc.), and a delicious Asian sauce (see Soy-Sriracha Stir-Fry Sauce, page 317). Eat this hot right out of the wok or cold as leftovers.

- **Weekly salads don't have to be boring!** Keep a large container of leafy greens washed, cut, and ready to eat in your refrigerator all week. A fan favorite is a mix of romaine and red leaf lettuce, or mix it up by adding baby kale, baby spinach, or a blend of mixed greens and arugula to keep it interesting. This makes it easy to have prepared salads throughout the week at dinners or to assemble a quick to-go lunch container to bring to work, school, or anywhere on the go. You can mix and match leftover protein (chicken, turkey, shrimp, hard-boiled eggs, etc.) with unlimited veggies. Toss in vinegar and extra-virgin olive oil or try the Goes with Everything Dressing (page 318) or Regal Lemon-Shallot Dressing (page 319) for a custom Cobb salad that turns out different each time.

In a Rush

There won't always be time to plan the week out perfectly. For those days that you're feeling particularly pressed for time, consider one of these options:

- **Buy salad kits.** Fresh, prepackaged salad kits can be found in the produce section of most grocery stores. Be sure to check the salad dressing—you may want to use your own if the one provided is too high in saturated fat. A good rule of thumb is to look for dressings with no more than 3 grams of saturated fat per serving. (We'll talk more about how to interpret nutrition facts labels later.)

- **Think green when you drink.** Throw a handful of spinach, arugula, or mixed greens into a smoothie for breakfast or an energizing snack. See part V for Key Lime Smoothie (page 251), Spinach and Coffee Protein Smoothie (page 252), and Strawberry Green Breakfast Smoothie (page 252).

- **Try a green add-on.** Add raw or sautéed greens to an omelet, sandwich, soup, or wrap.

OTHER VEGETABLES

Vegetables are so important for brain health and achieving a healthy weight that we put them on the list twice. First, as leafy green vegetables, and second, as what we call "other vegetables."

Other vegetables contain similar nutrients as leafy greens in varying amounts—important carotenoids such as beta-carotene and lutein that perform antioxidative and anti-inflammatory functions. A study conducted in the Netherlands observed people's fruit and vegetable intake over 5 years and compared their cognitive functioning. Vegetable intake was associated with slower decline of information and processing speed.[3] Additionally, other vegetables are excellent

---

MIND DIET TARGET

Add One Other — Go for Color

Aim for 1 serving of other colorful vegetables every day.

1 serving = ½ cup, cooked or raw

Examples: artichokes, asparagus, broccoli, brussels sprouts, cabbage, carrots, cauliflower, eggplant, green beans, leeks, mushrooms, okra, onions, peppers, pumpkin, snow peas, squash, sweet potatoes, tomatoes/tomato sauce, zucchini

---

for weight management, since they are high in fiber and water — two components that will create that feeling of fullness in the belly, trigger the release of leptin, and communicate the message to the brain that it is time to stop eating. Other vegetables contain an average of 25 calories per ½-cup serving, making them a great low-calorie option for achieving or maintaining a healthy weight. You can enhance the satiating effects of other vegetables by drinking a full glass of water with each meal and snack. Water's weight, combined with its expanded volume in the stomach, will help induce a quick feeling of fullness for zero additional calories.

WEIGHT LOSS ON THE MIND?

Incorporate plenty of high-fiber other vegetables to help you feel fuller faster and achieve your weight loss goals.

Other vegetables contain an average of 25 calories per ½-cup serving.

Drink a glass of water with each meal and snack to enhance the feeling of fullness.

The best indication of which vegetables are most nutritious is their color. The brightest and darkest vegetables typically carry the highest nutrient concentration. This is because the nutrients contained within the vegetables are supplying the plant with its pigment. For example, beta-carotene gives way to the orange pigment you see in carrots, bell peppers, pumpkins, and sweet potatoes; lycopene supplies tomatoes and tomato sauce with their deep red color; and a powerful antioxidant called anthocyanin is responsible for the beautiful purple found in the skin of the eggplant. Unfortunately, white potatoes don't count as other vegetables, since they are high in starchy carbohydrate without the benefit of the nutrient-rich pigment. The same goes for vegetable juices—these are typically too concentrated in sugars and often have a lot of added sodium as a preservative and flavor enhancer. As you continue to build your MINDful eating routine, add a splash of color to your vegetable choices to optimize brain health—the proof is in the pigment!

HOW TO ENJOY OTHER VEGETABLES

In a Routine

Add other vegetables to your leafy green salad for dinner or lunch.

- **Make veggie bites.** You can find most items already cut to bite-size in the grocery store, but if you don't want to invest in this luxury, you'll have to invest a little time instead. Peel and cut the carrots, slice the peppers, and cut the cucumbers into coins. Create raw veggie snack packs and store them in reusable containers or plastic bags for easy transport in a purse, briefcase, or backpack.

- **Make it airtight.** If your storage container is airtight, your veggies should stay fresh for a longer period of time. When moisture gets in, so does potential for spoilage.

- **Keep veggies in plain sight.** Store baby carrots, mini bell peppers, cucumber slices, and cherry tomatoes in the front of the refrigerator. Veggie drawers are great, but they're also often where our best-laid plans go to die—out of sight, out of mind! When produce begins to wilt, wrinkle, and turn dull, that's a clue that the nutritional value is declining.

- **Do a weekly salad prep.** Remember I mentioned that container of ready-to-eat leafy greens that keeps getting refreshed in my refrigerator each week? It sits next to two or three other containers filled with whatever other vegetables I have on hand. My family loves fresh red and orange bell peppers, cut into long, thin slices, so those are a weekly staple. The remaining veggies are determined based on leftovers from prepared meals or ingredients that didn't get used in other recipes. For example, let's say Monday's dinner is a chicken stir-fry with mixed vegetables, but an entire head each of cauliflower and broccoli is a lot more than needed to prepare the recipe. That means that the remaining broccoli and cauliflower will get cut up into smaller pieces and stored in containers to be used as added salad ingredients for the rest of the week.

- **Make your veggies mimic your junk food.** A few things make junk foods so tasty: texture, fat, sugar, and salt. Not everyone loves all those characteristics, but you may have an affinity for "crunchy-salty" flavors or perhaps you have more of a "sweet tooth." For example, if you're into crunchy-salty, you're probably drawn to potato chips, crackers, popcorn, pretzels, etc. You might instead try sprinkling a touch of sea salt on a mini red or orange bell pepper or on a bowl of sliced cucumbers and tomatoes for a quick salad. If you're lucky, sitting with that bowl of salty-crunchy will be just enough to trick your brain not to care whether you're eating veggies or potato chips! If you're not so lucky, try dipping, spreading, or sprinkling your veggies with balsamic vinegar, extra-virgin olive oil, hummus, jalapeño peppers (seeds = spice), lemon/lime/orange juice and/or zest, liquid aminos or low-sodium soy sauce, low-fat cottage cheese, nutritional yeast (vegan substitute for cheese), nut butter, salsa, yogurt-based dressings, crushed red or cayenne pepper, sriracha, or chili paste.

In a Routine other veggie snack examples are:

- Baby carrots + 1 to 2 tablespoons nut butter + cayenne pepper (optional)

- Tomato slices + ½ cup low-fat cottage cheese + ground black pepper + dried oregano

- Cucumber slices + pitted black or green olives + lemon juice + fresh or dried dill + black or crushed red pepper (optional), or with 2 tablespoons Garlicky Yogurt Sauce (page 315)

- Celery stalks + 1 to 2 tablespoons nut butter or Creamy Tahini Sauce (page 316) + 1 tablespoon fresh or frozen berries

- Mini bell peppers, carrot sticks, and snow peas (or any raw veggies) + 2 tablespoons hummus or Spicy Black Bean Hummus (page 300) or Arugula Pesto (page 314) or Creamy Spinach Dip (page 298)

- Cucumber coins topped with low-fat cottage cheese + lemon juice + fresh or dried dill and/or dried oregano

- Sliced tomatoes, cucumbers, and red onions + 1 table-spoon extra-virgin olive oil + 1½ teaspoons balsamic vinegar + dried oregano + chopped fresh parsley + sea salt + crushed red pepper (optional)

- **Follow four steps for veggie scraps.** Despite our best inten-tions, we often can't eat through our veggie supply quickly enough, so lots of scraps end up going bad in the fridge. Here are some ideas for extending the life of those veggies before the nutrients are all drained out of them:

Vegetables (Plural) and Fruit (Singular)

1. Choose your favorite fresh, frozen, or leftover "scrap" vegetables that you may not have used throughout the week or are at risk for going bad.

   o Bell peppers, broccoli, brussels sprouts, carrots, cauliflower, garlic, green beans, leafy greens (collards, mustard greens, kale, spinach, etc.), mushrooms, onions (red, yellow, white, etc.), tomatoes, zucchini

2. Add 1 to 2 tablespoons of healthy "sauce." The amount you'll use here is dependent upon the volume of your leftover veggies. A good rule of thumb is about 1 tablespoon sauce per 1 cup veggies.

   o Extra-virgin olive (best!), avocado, grapeseed, peanut, or canola oil; light salad dressing; liquid aminos or low-sodium soy sauce; balsamic vinegar; salsa; low-fat yogurt sauce; nutritional yeast

   o MIND sauces and dressings: Creamy Tahini Sauce (page 316), Balsamic Reduction (page 317), Goes with Everything Dressing (page 318), or Regal Lemon-Shallot Dressing (page 319)

3. Spice it up! Especially if your seasonings are salt-free, you should feel at liberty to use as much as you like—this is where the *real* flavor happens. Try some of these internationally inspired herbs and spices:

   o Italian (garlic, oregano, parsley, basil, rosemary, fennel)

   o Latin (cumin, paprika, jalapeño pepper, crushed red pepper, cilantro, lime)

   o East Asian (ginger, garlic, sesame seed, cloves)

   o Indian (curry, turmeric, celery seed, nutmeg, cinnamon)

   o Greek (onion powder, oregano, dill, basil, parsley, cumin, cloves, lemon)

4. Shake and stir-fry, bake, broil, or grill.

   ○ Toss everything into a large storage container or baggie, shake it up to distribute the sauce and seasonings, and cook over high heat for 10 to 30 minutes, until the veggies are crisp-tender.

If you have high blood pressure and are using salt as one of your add-ins to season your veggies, consider using salt-free herbs and spices instead.

You may be someone who prefers more bold flavors. The food industry creates many bold, flavorful products that contain ingredients high in salt and saturated fats such as oils, mayonnaise, cream, and butter. Citrus and spice are two great options to infuse bold flavors without all the sodium and saturated fat. Try fresh lemon, lime, and orange juices and grated zest. If you like heat, try crushed red or cayenne pepper, sriracha, or chili paste. Salsas come in a variety of spice levels and are low-calorie. Try yogurt-based dressings, balsamic vinegar, low-sodium soy sauce or liquid aminos (for the taste of salt with less sodium), and nutritional yeast (a great substitute for cheese without the saturated fat).

In a Rush

When you're in a hurry, vegetables are typically the first food to get sacrificed. A common misconception is that vegetables are boring and take too long to prepare to make them taste good. My recommendation is to add vegetables to things that are convenient and tasty. Remember, the goal isn't to eat perfectly. You're not on a diet. You're trying to find opportunities to maximize your intake of brain-healthy foods and limit your intake of brain-harmful foods. Here are some ideas:

- **Use veggies as fillers.** Bulk up soups, chili, and stir-fries with your favorite vegetables. This is a great way to get in veggies, while also amping up the flavor and nutrients in your soups or stir-fries. Cooking methods like boiling are not ideal for preserving nutrients unless you plan to consume the water, as in a soup. Dry-heat methods like baking, broiling, roasting, stir-frying, sautéing, or steaming/braising are best. In some cases the nutrient composition actually increases when the vegetable is cooked — this is true for lycopene in tomatoes and beta-carotene in carrots.

- **Consider frozen veggies.** Fresh veggies are good, but sometimes your faves may not be in season, or the refrigerator veggie drawer may have claimed victory again. Frozen veggies can be even better since they are frozen at peak ripeness, preserving the nutrient content. Add frozen veggies to soups, salads, sandwiches, or even on top of Friday night pizza.

- **Look for healthy frozen meals.** I think frozen meals get a bad rap. Most people associate these meals with high sodium levels; however, when comparing these meals to restaurant and other convenience foods consumed away from the home, many of them can be much healthier. I recommend looking for three components on a frozen meal package:

  1. Check to see if the volume of food is made up of a significant amount of vegetables. Half of the container would be great, but at least one-quarter is key. If a meal does not contain enough veggies, you can toss some right into the meal container. Typically, there's enough sauce in those meals, and veggies like broccoli or brussels sprouts do a great job of soaking up all the deliciousness to make the meal a little heartier and healthier.

  2. Choose meals with no more than 600 milligrams sodium.

  3. Aim for no more than 3 grams of saturated fat for the whole meal.

BERRIES

Perhaps the most distinguishing characteristic of the MIND diet compared to all other healthy dietary patterns is the recommendation to focus on only one fruit category: berries.

MIND DIET TARGET

BERRY All Other Fruits

Aim for 5 servings of berries each week.

1 serving = ½ cup

Examples: blackberries, blueberries, raspberries, strawberries

---

The most predominant nutrient in berries is a polyphenol flavonoid called anthocyanin, responsible for protecting cells against oxidative injury, shielding vulnerable neurons, and enhancing function of existing neuronal structures in the brain. Berries are rich in vitamin C, a powerful antioxidant and a facilitator of iron absorption in the body. The latter function is particularly useful for anyone who may have issues with iron-deficiency anemia. That means combining berries with a meal can help the body absorb more iron from plant-based "non-heme" iron food sources, such as leafy green vegetables, beans, nuts, and whole grains.

Data from the Nurses' Health Study, one of the largest investigations of chronic disease health risks in women spanning more than 40 years, suggests that high intakes of blueberries and strawberries could delay cognitive aging by up to 2½ years.[4] These results validated earlier work from the same group that showed just 2 or more servings of berries per week helped improve diminishing physical functioning, thinking capabilities, and mental health.[5] The same pattern was observed in both men and women in the CHAP and MAP studies, which was then translated to risk for development of disease. People who ate berries twice a week had a 32 percent reduction in risk for development of Alzheimer's disease. In a later study that explored the actual brain pathology markers of Alzheimer's disease, a bioactive in strawberries called pelargonidin was associated with lower levels of phosphorylated tau tangles, suggesting that strawberries in particular may play a powerful role in reducing risk for Alzheimer's disease.[6]

Another "berry good" quality of our fruity flavonoid friends is that they are the absolute best fruit you can eat for weight management. We often hear that a healthy diet consists of "fruits and vegetables." In terms of macronutrient composition, berries and all other fruits technically fall in the carbohydrate group. However, for the purposes of the MIND diet, we are going to put berries with the leafy greens and other vegetables. This is another reminder to think of berries separate from all other fruits and the first invitation to think of other fruits separate from vegetables.

A key message I've been trying to drum into my clients over the past 20 years—not just for brain health but also for weight loss—is that fruits and vegetables are *not* created equal. As stated previously, berries were shown to be the only fruit to have an impact on brain health.[7] And for my clients seeking weight loss, berries are typically the only fruit I recommend eating in high amounts. This is because compared to other fruits, berries are the highest in fiber and the lowest in sugar, making them more likely to be filling and satisfying, rather than spiking blood sugar levels and leaving you feeling hungry.

WEIGHT LOSS ON THE MIND?

Compared to all other fruits, berries are the highest in fiber and the lowest in sugar, making them a great choice when trying to achieve or maintain a healthy weight.

HOW TO ENJOY BERRIES

In a Routine

All varieties of berries count when it comes to the MIND diet, and frozen are just as good as fresh, since they're frozen at the peak of freshness, so the valuable nutrients remain intact. In fact, for the MIND trial, participants were given frozen blueberries to help them achieve 5 servings per week. We do *not* recommend counting dried berries such as dried cranberries as a MIND food serving. Similar to vegetable juice, dried berries are concentrated and thus tend to be much higher in sugar, and they have not been shown in research studies to be connected to brain health like whole berries. My first recommendation is to always keep frozen berries on hand. You'd be surprised by the plethora of things you can do with frozen berries:

- **Drink berrywater.** Add ½ cup frozen berries to a glass of water and keep in the fridge for a refreshing beverage. A few lemon wedges and mint leaves can make this a party favorite!

- **Start your day with grainberry.** Cook your oatmeal, grits, or cream of wheat with ½ cup frozen berries for a flavored variety of your morning staple.

- **Cook up an easy berry chutney.** In a small saucepan, heat ½ tablespoon extra-virgin olive oil, 2 tablespoons diced shallot, ½ cup frozen berries, and a splash of dry red wine. Stir and simmer to make a sauce. Use as a chutney over chicken, turkey, or fish.

- **Make berry syrup.** Heat ½ cup frozen berries in a small saucepan until they burst and create a sauce. Use as "syrup" over pancakes and waffles instead of maple or commercial syrups.

- **Have berries for dessert.** This could not be simpler — really. Portion out ½ cup frozen berries. Eat. Repeat. You won't believe what a treat this is until you try it. An old Weight-Watchers trick is to do the same with frozen grapes — but berries are so much healthier!

- **Do a berry transfer.** Each night, transfer ½ cup frozen berries from the freezer to the refrigerator. The next day, use in the same way you would fresh berries.

If you're not willing to embrace your inner creative to get into a routine love affair with frozen berries, and you have the means to go fresh year-round, I recommend simply making it a habit to add ½ cup berries to a meal or snack on most days. It might be easiest to do this with breakfast to ensure you check it off your list. The goal is five ½-cup servings per week, so you can take the weekends off to indulge in a more decadent breakfast experience, take a break from berries, or take a break from breakfast and sleep in!

In a Rush

Whether you're choosing fresh or frozen, here are a few quick and easy ways to incorporate berries:

- **Blend a morning protein "bluethie."** Combine ½ cup blueberries (or any berries), 1 cup low-fat milk or soy milk, and 1 serving whey protein powder in a blender, blend well, and enjoy!

- **Serve up a breakfast side.** Serve ½ cup berries with any breakfast as a side — beside your eggs and toast, beside your avocado toast, or sprinkled on your oatmeal, yogurt, or cereal.

- **Get the snacktime blues.** For an afternoon snack, ½ cup blueberries (or any berries) goes great with a handful of almonds, a low-fat cheese stick, or a cup of Greek yogurt.

CHAPTER 9

Unsaturated Fats: Extra-Virgin Olive Oil, Nuts, and Seeds

The MIND diet foods categorized as unsaturated fats include extra-virgin olive oil (EVOO) and nuts and seeds (Nut).

Unsaturated Fats		MIND Food Points	
Extra-Virgin Olive Oil (EVOO) **Goal:** 2 servings/day **Serving size:** 1 tablespoon		0–6 servings/week	0
		7–13 servings/week	0.5
		14+ servings/week	1
Nuts & Seeds (Nut) **Goal:** 5 servings/week **Serving size:** 1 ounce nuts or seeds or 2 tablespoons nut/seed butter		0 servings/week	0
		1–4 servings/week	0.5
		5+ servings/week	1

Dietary fats are crucial because they help the body absorb and transport important nutrients, provide a concentrated source of energy to the body, and offer a great amount of sensory appeal in terms of enhancing the taste and smell of foods. Fats fall into one of three different types, with varying degree of functionality and usefulness in the body. They are also the most calorically dense macronutrient, providing 9 calories per gram. The American Heart Association names these three types of fat the good, the bad, and the ugly, as described in the following table.

FATS AND THEIR FUNCTION[1]

	THE GOOD	THE BAD	THE UGLY
FAT	**Monounsaturated & Polyunsaturated Fatty Acids (MUFAs & PUFAs)**	**Saturated Fats**	**Trans Fats & Hydrogenated Oils**
FUNCTION	Lowers LDL (bad cholesterol) Lowers risk for heart disease and stroke	Increases LDL (bad cholesterol) Increases risk for heart disease and stroke	Increases LDL (bad cholesterol) Lowers HDL (good cholesterol) Increases risk for heart disease and stroke Increases risk for type 2 diabetes
FOOD SOURCES	**MIND Foods to Choose:** extra-virgin olive oil, nuts (such as walnuts), seeds (such as flaxseed and sunflower seeds), fatty fish (such as salmon, tuna, herring, lake trout, mackerel, and sardines) **Other Foods to Choose in Moderation:** avocados, oils (such as canola, safflower, and sesame)	**MIND Foods to Limit:** red/processed meats, full-fat cheese, butter, fried foods, sweets and pastries **Other Foods to Avoid:** fat from chicken/pork, coconut oil, palm kernel, palm oil	**MIND Foods to Limit:** sweets and pastries, stick margarine, fried foods **Other Foods to Avoid:** processed foods made with partially hydrogenated oils

EXTRA-VIRGIN OLIVE OIL

A well-known MVP of the Mediterranean diet that remains a key component in the MIND diet is extra-virgin olive oil (EVOO).

MIND DIET TARGET

EVOOlutionize Your Cooking

Aim for 2 servings of EVOO each day.

1 serving = 1 tablespoon

Unrefined extra-virgin olive oil

The MIND diet researchers found in their CHAP and MAP studies that those who used extra-virgin olive oil as the primary oil compared to other vegetable oils had a reduced risk for developing Alzheimer's disease. EVOO is rich in monounsaturated fatty acids (MUFAs). It is well established that MUFAs can help lower LDL cholesterol, thus reducing one's risk for heart disease and stroke. It was more recently discovered that these good-for-you fats can also help regulate irregular heartbeat patterns and supply blood and nutrients to the brain to improve neurotransmission and contribute to brain health. EVOO is also rich in polyphenols and vitamin E, protecting cells against oxidative injury and inflammation. Vitamin E is thought to be one of the components that protects the brain from accumulation of beta-amyloid plaques, the hallmark protein of Alzheimer's disease.

HOW TO ENJOY EXTRA-VIRGIN OLIVE OIL

EVOO that is "unrefined" has been naturally extracted from olives without additional chemicals or heat. This keeps the acid levels low and preserves the beneficial MUFAs and antioxidants, while producing a more robust aroma and flavor. That's why if you've ever had EVOO overseas, or from a high-end grocery store or restaurant, it probably tasted extra good.

If you're shopping on a budget, my advice is to keep your eye out for sales on the good stuff. Look for certification seals such as the ones pictured below to be sure the manufacturers followed standardized protocols to produce the highest quality product and not just empty calories.

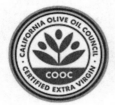 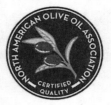

Remember, the goal for EVOO is 2 tablespoons per day, which is equivalent to 240 calories. To put that into perspective, if you add 250 calories to your diet without balancing those calories with either a swap of another food or increased exercise, you could gain ½ pound per week. In other words, you want to make sure that the addition of your EVOO is worth the energy—quite literally!

WEIGHT LOSS ON THE MIND?

Although EVOO is important for brain health, it is also dense in calories. If you are working toward a weight loss goal, be MINDful of the portions for this MIND food.

Aim for 2 servings/day.
1 serving = 1 tablespoon

Cooking with EVOO

Getting into a routine for making EVOO a regular part of your diet means rethinking how you use added fats in your meals—you need to EVOOlutionize your cooking. And step one is to be MINDful of the way you cook with it. As news about the health benefits of olive oil began to emerge, more of my patients began to tell me they were using EVOO for cooking. And I witnessed it firsthand in our lifestyle groups and cooking programs. People were also taking what I call the "more is better" approach by pouring EVOO over salads to create a swimming pool of mixed leafy greens, filling the bottom of the pan with EVOO and then turning the burners up to high heat as if we were getting ready to deep-fry their brussels sprouts, and slathering the salmon fillets until they almost slid off the baking sheet before putting them into a 425°F oven. This is not the healthiest approach, since EVOO is high in calories, and some research suggests that it shouldn't be used in high-heat cooking for extended periods of time.[2] We used to think this was because it was not "heat stable," meaning that above low-medium heat, the fats oxidize or become damaged. Just as we don't want our brain cells or any other cells to oxidize and become damaged, we do not want the fats in our foods to become damaged.

Research has emerged recently to suggest that it *is* safe to cook with EVOO. A group in Australia studied a variety of cooking oils to determine if the smoke point of an oil was the only factor that contributed to its breakdown under high heat.[3] When EVOO was evaluated, it was found that because of the high concentration of vitamin E and presence of polyunsaturated fatty acids (PUFAs), both powerful antioxidants that protect against cell breakdown, the oil remained stable and therefore safe to cook with.

All that being said, we recommend making it a habit to use your EVOO *most often* in its natural, raw form, and if you do cook with it, try not to heat it above medium cooking temperatures and be MIND-ful of the amount you use.

Below is a list of high-quality EVOOs based on beneficial fatty acid and polyphenol content:

- Kirkland Signature organic, Newman's Own organic, Bertolli, Colavita, California Olive Ranch, Trader Joe's Premium, 365, Pompeian, Lucini Premium Select, Simply Nature organic, Cibaria organic, Star, La Tourangelle

In a Routine

- **Mix up a weekly salad dressing.** As you may have guessed, my containers of leafy greens and other veggies don't get assembled into delicious salads without dressings to make them complete. I also make salad dressings in advance each week. I use dressing containers to mix my dressing on my meal prep day, shake and pour as needed, and put back into the refrigerator for the rest of the week. If you're making your dressing with EVOO (highly recommended!), you'll want to remember that since it's an unsaturated fat, it doesn't become liquid until it gets to room temperature, so you may want to take the dressing container out of the fridge for 10 or 20 minutes before you're ready to pour it onto the salad.

- **Marinate your veggies.** Whether you've gotten into a routine of following the four steps for veggie scraps (see page 68) or you already have a favorite way to cook your veggies, you don't need a pool of oil to make them taste good or to cook them well. First, to keep EVOO intake at the right level so that you get the right dose of beneficial brain nutrients without overdoing the calories, I suggest incorporating a marinade to help flavor your food. Try the Garlicky Yogurt Sauce (page 315), Balsamic Reduction (page 317), or Goes with Everything Dressing (page 318). If you tend to prefer saucier dishes, you can combine EVOO with low-calorie ingredients such as lemon or lime juice, low-sodium soy sauce, or liquid aminos for those watching sodium intake. And, as always, the real joy is buried in the herbs and spices—load 'em up! See page 68 if you need help with flavor combos.

- **Make a trade.** Remember that since EVOO is dense in calories, the incorporation of 2 tablespoons a day will likely require getting into the habit of swapping out something else, since we should be MINDful that being overweight is another risk factor for Alzheimer's disease. Additionally, we know that mono- and polyunsaturated fats can aid in a healthy shift of cholesterol profiles when those are used as a substitute for saturated and trans fats. So, it's important to think about what you can trade out when incorporating EVOO. Instead of topping bread and toast with butter, consider dipping them in portioned EVOO; add EVOO to cooked vegetables and pasta or rice instead of butter, cheese, or alfredo sauces; use it as a substitute for creams in soup and casserole recipes; or make homemade dips with EVOO instead of buying store-bought products like hummus, pesto, and tomato sauces. See the chapter on Sauces and Toppers (page 314).

- **Say no to EVOO for fatty fish.** Believe it or not, you do not need to add EVOO or any additional oil or fat to fatty fish such as salmon, tuna, mackerel, herring, lake trout, sardines, or anchovies. I think people have gotten into the habit of greasing the pan or coating their meat before cooking without understanding why. Is it to enhance the cooking process? For health benefits? In the case of these fish, no additional fat is needed—that's why they are called "fatty" fish. They contain the beneficial mono- and polyunsaturated fats that provide brain and heart health benefits.

  - **Exception to the rule.** If you're seeking flavor through added fat, such as in a marinade, be MINDful of the amount you are using and consider combining it with the lower-calorie ingredients mentioned above. See Broiled Arctic Char (page 268) and Chickpea Tuna Salad (page 273).

In a Rush

Out of all 10 MIND diet foods, EVOO was probably the most difficult for our team of dietitians in the MIND study to come up with creative ideas for getting 2 tablespoons in each day while maintaining the goal of weight loss. Kudos to our research participants for their brilliant (and entertaining!) ideas:

- Roz, one of our MIND trial participants, liked to get in her 2 tablespoons a day by dipping her fresh whole-grain bread into EVOO as a midday snack. She discovered the perfect measuring tool to be a shot glass. She only needed to measure the EVOO once into the shot glass to see that the line etched on the side told her exactly where to stop (1½ fluid ounces just happens to be equivalent to 2 tablespoons). Some people have a midday shot of whiskey, but Roz was drunk with happiness over her daily shot of EVOO.

- Other ways to get in 2 tablespoons of EVOO when in a rush include blending it into a smoothie, spooning it on a bowl of oatmeal, spreading it on toast instead of butter, or even dolloping it into your favorite soup.

NUTS AND SEEDS

Another set of key players on the Mediterranean diet that continue to occupy the brain-nourishing spotlight on the MIND diet are nuts (including nut/seed butters) and seeds.

MIND DIET TARGET

MIND NUTrition

Aim for 5 servings of nuts/seeds or nut/seed butter each week.

1 serving = 1 ounce nuts/seeds or 2 tablespoons nut/seed butter

Examples: nuts such as almonds, walnuts, cashews, peanuts, pistachios; peanut butter or other nut butters; seeds such as pumpkin, chia, flax, sunflower, hemp; seed butters such as sunflower

---

Nuts are rich sources of omega-3 fatty acids (specifically, alpha-linolenic acid, or ALA). Just like EVOO, these unsaturated fats carry blood and nutrients to the brain and heart, improving neurotransmission and regulating heart rhythms. Again, like EVOO, nuts are antioxidant powerhouses, packed with polyphenols and vitamin E to protect cells against oxidative injury and inflammation and potentially prevent buildup of harmful beta-amyloid plaques in the brain. In the PREDIMED study, people who followed the Mediterranean diet enhanced with walnuts were found to have reduced risk for coronary heart disease and demonstrated marked improvements in their cognitive abilities.[4] Walnuts and almonds are the most nutrient-dense, but we recommend all nuts as part of a brain-healthy and heart-healthy eating pattern.

Seeds, such as sunflower, chia, hemp, and flax, contain many of the same beneficial brain- and heart-healthy nutrients as nuts; therefore, these foods also make it onto the MIND diet's list. As always, be MINDful of portions since seeds are also very calorie-dense.

If you have a nut allergy, the best thing to do is to avoid this category altogether (including seeds due to potential cross-contamination)—stay safe! Remember that the beauty of the MIND diet is that you do not have to get a perfect score on each individual food in order to get a total MIND diet score that represents moderate risk reduction for Alzheimer's disease. If you're avoiding nuts, think about what other foods on the list might make up for those missed points. The best place to start would be to ensure you're getting in all your EVOO servings, since it falls into the larger category of unsaturated fats and contains similar nutrients as nuts. Fatty fish (more on this later) also contains unsaturated fats. Another important nutrient in nuts is healthy protein, also plentiful in fish and poultry, making these good options if you are unable to consume nuts.

HOW TO ENJOY NUTS AND SEEDS

In a Routine

- **Be a smart nut shopper.** My first recommendation is to be choosy about which products you purchase.

  - Raw, unsalted nuts will always be the best choice, since that means minimal processing and therefore minimal opportunity for the beneficial nutrients to be depleted. If you don't have to worry about blood pressure issues or are a highly active person who needs the additional salt, then lightly salted may be okay for you.

  - Avoid honey-roasted or other flavored varieties of nuts. Not only will their nutrients be diminished through processing, but they will likely have added sugars, salt, and other chemical flavor enhancers.

  - "Nuts" should be the first ingredient on the list. Why should anything else make up the largest percentage of a product that is supposed to be nuts or nut butter? *Hint:* It shouldn't.

- **Follow snack portion NUTrition.** Another thing our nutty friends have in common with EVOO is caloric density. A 1-ounce serving is equivalent to about ¼ cup nuts or 2 tablespoons nut/seed butter, or about 200 calories, depending upon the nut or butter. Although the MIND diet goal for the nut group is not a daily one, keep in mind that if you're looking to lose weight, you should reduce your daily intake by about 250 calories a day, which may mean swapping out 200 or so calories from some other food or drink source in order to fit in your weekly dose of nut nutrients without busting your calorie budget. One idea is to preportion five snack-size containers of nuts every week.

- **Try some nutty recipes.** There's no need to plan ahead for elaborate recipes. Nuts are a great topping for just about anything. Crush up walnuts, almonds, or cashews and use as toppings for salad, fish, yogurt, or even a bowl of fresh mixed fruit. Nut butters are a great use for binding foods or adding texture and creaminess. You can find great recipe ideas in part V, such as Hippie Oat Bowls (page 247), Chia Seed Pudding with Berries (page 250), Strawberry Green Breakfast Smoothie (page 252), Arugula Hemp Seed Salad (page 292), Protein Power Bites (page 308), and Toasted Nuts (page 321).

WEIGHT LOSS ON THE MIND?

Be MINDful of portions for nuts if you are working toward a weight loss goal. There are about 200 calories in 1 serving.

Aim for 5 servings per week.
1 serving = 1 ounce nuts or 2 tablespoons nut/seed butter

In a Rush

- **Have a quick schmear.** Nut/seed butters are some of the best foods to eat when in a hurry, since they are so portable. It's really easy to schmear a couple of tablespoons of nut butter onto a slice of whole-grain toast; a pinch of ground cinnamon on top makes for a delightful breakfast or a quick snack on the run. Nut butter also goes well with a few whole-grain crackers for a midday snack, or over a ½ banana or an apple before going for a walk. Another idea that surprises people is dipping baby carrots into mini to-go cups of peanut butter. Nut butter and carrots sounds like an odd combo, but the sweetness of the carrots combined with the savory taste of the nut butter is quite tasty! Lastly, a spoonful of nut butter on a celery stalk brings me back to my childhood. We used to throw a few raisins on top and call this Ants on a Log!

- **Try nut bars.** I'm not a huge fan of snack or meal-replacement bars, since many of them are highly processed and really just glorified candy bars. That being said, they are incredibly portable and when you're in a time-crunched situation, a bar can certainly be a great way to stave off hunger until you can get your next balanced meal—that is, *if* it meets some key criteria. Look for bars that have at least 5 grams of protein, no more than 3 grams of saturated fat, and no more than 10 grams of sugar.

  Here are some brands I like—but *please read the food label!* One of my goals is to teach you *how* to eat, rather than have you be dependent upon a written list that may become obsolete with the perpetually changing food product market. Keep in mind, in order for the bar to count on the list as a full serving of nuts, it must contain ¼ cup nuts—that's likely about half of the volume of the bar. So, if some type of nut isn't listed as the first or second ingredient, it probably won't count as a MIND food.

  - RXBar, Kind Protein, OWYN, Built, GoMacro, Think, Clif Protein, Quest, Luna Protein, Naked Nutrition, Pure Protein

CHAPTER 10

Proteins: Fish, Seafood, and Poultry

Protein foods break down into amino acids, the building blocks needed to preserve the integrity of hair, skin, nails, muscles, and many important hormones in the body. Protein is one of the three macronutrient groups, and it provides energy and helps fill you up and make you feel satisfied. Dietary proteins provide 4 calories per gram and play an important role in brain health. A study using data from the National Health and Nutrition Examination Survey (NHANES 2011–2014) showed that older adults who consumed greater amounts of protein demonstrated better cognitive functioning compared to those with lower protein intakes.[1] According to the Centers for Disease Control and Prevention, subjective cognitive decline (SCD) is a measure in which people self-report confusion or memory loss, and it is thought to be one of the earliest noticeable symptoms of Alzheimer's disease and related dementias. A study using data from the Nurses' Health Study and the Health Professionals Follow-Up Study between 2008 and 2012 explored the role of protein and SCD and found that intake from lean protein sources such as white-meat poultry, fish, and beans/legumes was associated with lower SCD, while intake from protein foods with higher saturated fat content such as hot dogs was associated with higher SCD. This suggests that the *type of protein* we eat is important when it comes to brain health.[2]

FISH AND SEAFOOD

The first type of protein on the MIND diet is fish and seafood (Fsh).

MIND DIET TARGET

Go Fish

Consume fish and seafood once weekly.

1 serving = 3 to 5 ounces

Highest in DHA: albacore tuna, anchovies, mackerel, salmon, sardines

Other good choices: clams, cod, halibut, lobster, mahi-mahi, oysters, scallops, shrimp, tilapia

---

Both the American Heart Association and the Mediterranean diet guidelines recommend consumption of fish at least twice weekly. Fatty fish (such as salmon, albacore tuna, mackerel, sardines, and anchovies) provides the brain with beneficial polyunsaturated fats similar to those in nuts, but the omega-3s are in the form of docosahexaenoic acid (DHA). The omega-3s act by nourishing the brain with blood and nutrients, improving neurotransmission. We know that these nutrients can reduce risk for heart disease and stroke, too, through lowering LDL cholesterol. Fish containing omega-3s may also help prevent depression. A review of studies including more than 150,000 people found that individuals who consumed fish regularly were 20 percent less likely to experience depression, highlighting another important part of cognitive health: emotional health and well-being.[3]

For brain health, all sources of fish and seafood were shown to provide benefits, not just those high in omega-3 fatty acids. It was found that eating as little as 1 serving a week was sufficient to prevent cognitive decline.[4]

Fish and seafood are also rich in B vitamins, such as B_6 and B_{12}, which are essential for proper functioning in the brain, protection from oxidation and inflammation, and growth of new DNA. And finally, many fish contain tryptophan, an amino acid essential for production of serotonin and melatonin in the brain, which are connected to memory and learning.

HOW TO ENJOY FISH AND SEAFOOD

In a Routine

Getting into the habit to "go fish" once a week simply requires identifying your fish and seafood for the week, planning a cooking method, and keeping it interesting by experimenting with different toppings or sides with the main dish. The choice of fish and seafood will likely be dependent upon what's in season in your geographic location and whatever is available at your local grocer. I recommend looking for specials at the grocery store or visiting specialty fish and seafood markets if possible for the freshest options at the best prices.

For recipes, see Laura's fish and seafood creations in part V: Fancy Smoked Salmon Toast (page 246), Broiled Arctic Char (page 268), Poached Salmon with Toasted Almonds and Parsley (page 270), Pasta with Marinated Tomatoes and Shrimp (page 271), Chickpea Tuna Salad (page 273), and White Fish with Olives and Artichokes (page 275).

In a Rush

Since the goal is to consume fish and seafood only once a week, it should be relatively easy to get in your 3 to 5 ounces. If you don't have time to shop and prepare the fresh options, know that many canned and frozen products are available, such as canned tuna, salmon, clams, and mussels and frozen shrimp and fillets of salmon and white fish. Steer toward products canned in water and frozen products without added sauces. Also be sure to check the label and aim for 600 milligrams or less of sodium for your fish and seafood meals if you have high blood pressure.

AVOIDING FISH AND SEAFOOD

If you have a true allergy to fish and seafood, particularly shellfish, please stay safe and avoid it. If it's a matter of preference, however, or if you're thinking of experimenting with a vegetarian diet as a new approach, I'd like to invite you to consider having an open mind when it comes to trying out different types of fish and seafood options. Over the years of working with people, I have observed a common theme when it comes to preferences — or perceived preferences — around fish and seafood. Many people have tried one type of fish or seafood and then decided that they don't like *any* of it. This is like saying that you don't like the beach you went to as a kid, therefore you don't like any beaches at all. But there are so many different types of beaches — sand, rock, on a lake, near the mountains, etc. Wouldn't it depend on where you'd like to go, what you'd like to eat, and what activities you enjoy? The same is true for fish and seafood. There are so many different types, and preference will depend on the texture, temperature, preparation method, and even the social atmosphere.

Another reason people may avoid fish and seafood is fear of mercury toxicity. All fish and seafood are exposed to some mercury due to pollution of oceans, rivers, and lakes or from mercury in ocean sediment. However, national guidelines from the Food and Drug Administration, Environmental Protection Agency, and American Heart Association agree that the benefits outweigh the risks when considering fish consumption for both heart and brain health benefits, especially at the recommended levels of 1 or 2 servings per week (a total of 6 to 10 ounces). Fish that contain the highest concentrations of mercury tend to be shark, swordfish, king mackerel, tilefish, and albacore tuna. The recommendation is for women who are pregnant or breastfeeding and young children to avoid these varieties, but to increase consumption of lower-mercury fish and seafood to support maternal health and fetal growth and development.[5]

We got a lot of questions in the MIND trial about whether it would be acceptable to skip the fish and seafood category or take a fish oil supplement for people who did not care for fish and seafood. There is some evidence to support the positive effects of omega-3 intake in supplement form for cognition,[6] but the consensus in the field of experts, including the Global Council on Brain Health (GCBH), is that it is much better to get these nutrients from food versus supplements. The GCBH is a diverse group of scientists, health professionals, educators, and policy advocates convened by the American Association of Retired People (AARP) who are experts in brain health and cognition; they carefully and objectively review all the available evidence, including the risks and benefits of implementing recommendations. For all supplements marketed toward brain health, including fish oil and other products containing omega-3 fatty acids, the council states, "We do not endorse any ingredient, product, or supplement formulation specifically for brain health, unless your health care provider has identified that you have a specific nutrient deficiency."[7]

They go on to say that some of these supplements may actually be harmful if taken in excess or if they interact with prescribed medications. I remember Dr. Morris being wary of many of the supplement studies that demonstrated positive outcomes, since they were often done with people who were deficient in the nutrients being tested. Indeed, if you have a nutrient deficiency, you could and should expect to see an improvement as a result of supplementation. It would be important to confirm with your doctor and then supplement accordingly in that case. But the message that supplementation is beneficial for all individuals, even those who are likely *not* deficient, is inaccurate and could even be harmful.

Just as in the case of nuts, it is perfectly possible to get a therapeutic MIND diet score without the fish and seafood category. However, we want to encourage you to reap the benefits of *all* of the categories, especially since the DHA omega-3 fatty acids found in fatty fish are one of the "essential" brain nutrients, so we encourage any non–fish and seafood eaters to be open-minded about integrating these foods into your lifestyle (notwithstanding allergies, of course!). Or at least lean in with an attitude of curiosity.

> "I tend to approach everything I do with an extreme sense of curiosity. I'm just so curious about everything…it's fun! Approach it with a sense of curiosity, it's a much easier way of life than one would think. It's much more than a diet…it's a way of life."
>
> —*Rosalyn L.*

POULTRY

We recommend having 2 or more 3- to 5-ounce servings per week of poultry (Poul). This is roughly equivalent to the recommendations in the Mediterranean and DASH diets. Poultry is a low-fat source of protein that carries a good amount of the brain-healthy B vitamins. It's also a source of tryptophan, an essential amino acid that's converted into the neurotransmitter serotonin in the brain, which helps regulate sleep, mood, and appetite. Some examples of plant sources of tryptophan are soybeans, sesame seeds, and sunflower seeds. In the CHAP study, it was found that eating foods with both the B vitamin niacin and tryptophan was associated with slower rates of cognitive decline.[8] For the MIND diet, choose skinless white-meat chicken and turkey for your poultry meals.

MIND DIET TARGET

Chicken "Meats" Turkey

Consume poultry twice weekly.

1 serving = 3 to 5 ounces

Examples: skinless white-meat (breast) chicken or turkey (not fried), deli-style chicken or turkey, ground chicken or turkey

---

HOW TO ENJOY POULTRY

In a Routine

- **Get out your slow cooker!** Rotate your favorite poultry dishes from week to week and make enough for leftovers. In my house, we make chicken tacos almost every week. It couldn't be easier! Put 1 pound of boneless, skinless chicken breasts into a slow cooker, along with a 16-ounce container of salsa or pico de gallo (we like ours fresh from the deli), a drained 15-ounce can of whole kernel corn (frozen works, too), and 1 envelope of taco seasoning. Cover and set to cook on low for 6 to 8 hours. I shred the chicken meat about midway through the cook time and then throw it back in to soak up the rest of the delicious juices. For low-sodium, skip the seasoning envelope and add your own spices, such as chili powder, ground cumin, paprika, black pepper, garlic powder, onion powder, and crushed red pepper. Enjoy with corn or whole-grain flour tortillas, shredded lettuce, sliced black olives, fresh cilantro, and lime wedges. If you like, sprinkle with low-fat shredded cheese and add a dollop of nonfat plain Greek yogurt (instead of sour cream).

- **Transform your weekly salad into a meal.** Let's go back to those containers of leafy greens and other veggies I recommended you have ready and waiting in the fridge for easy access. Use leftover chicken from other meals or store-bought cooked chicken chunks or strips as the main ingredient on top of your weekly salad for a complete lunch or dinner. Simply toss with vinegar and EVOO or try Goes with Everything Dressing (page 318) or Regal Lemon-Shallot Dressing (page 319).

- **Stash a bird in the freezer.** Keep boneless, skinless chicken breasts and lean ground turkey or chicken (at least 93 percent lean) stocked in the freezer to ensure you don't run out of healthy protein options.

- **Poultry fatigue?** Many people complain that they are tired of the same chicken and turkey recipes and want something new. Check out Laura's poultry recipes in part V—there's no shortage of creativity in these novel dishes! Turkish Tabbouleh with Chicken Meatballs (page 254), Grilled Chicken Spiedies (page 256), Roast Chicken (page 265), and Spaghetti Squash Bolognese (page 267) are just a few examples.

In a Rush

- **Pick up a rotisserie chicken.** This is the "SOS" of dinnertime in our house when we don't have a plan and don't want to resort to eating out. It's so simple to grab a bird (or two, depending on its size and how many people you're feeding) from the local grocery store, perfectly roasted, hot, and ready to enjoy. This protein can get paired with any veggie and/or grain for the dinner meal, and leftovers can be used the next day as a quick protein option on top of salads, inside sandwiches or wraps, in chicken salad mixtures, or even as an added component of a soup to boost the protein. For the most brain and heart protection, remove the skin and stick with the white meat portions of the bird.

- **Make a quick chicken salad.** Combine canned, leftover, or rotisserie chicken with plain nonfat Greek yogurt (instead of mayo), chopped celery, red onions, dried dill, Dijon mustard, and fresh lemon juice in a bowl and mix. Enjoy with whole-grain crackers and/or sliced fresh veggies.

- **Don't forget burgers.** Store turkey or chicken patties in individual containers in the freezer. They take only a few minutes to thaw and cook, then just pair with a whole-grain bun; add lettuce, tomatoes, onions, pickles, and any of your other favorite burger toppings.

PROTEIN AND WEIGHT LOSS

In this program, we will encourage you to think of both the fish and seafood and poultry categories as protein foods.

Proteins	MIND Food Points	
Fish & Seafood (Fsh) **Goal:** 1 serving/week **Serving size:** 3–5 ounces	0 servings/week	0
	1+ servings/week	1
Poultry (Poul) **Goal:** 2 servings/week **Serving size:** 3–5 ounces without skin/bones	0 servings/week	0
	1 serving/week	0.5
	2+ servings/week	1

Researchers have been studying the role of protein in weight loss for decades. A review article published in the *American Journal of Clinical Nutrition* conclusively demonstrated the benefits of higher protein (greater than 25 percent of total calories) versus lower protein as a component of weight loss diets, resulting in the following:

- Greater weight loss

- Greater fat mass loss

- Preservation of lean body mass (that is, less muscle breakdown)

- Reduction in inches around the waist

- Improvements in cardiovascular risk markers such as blood pressure and triglycerides

The mechanisms thought to be responsible for protein's ability to produce these benefits include an increase in the feeling of fullness and satiety hormones, thereby reducing energy intake and modulation of energy metabolism.[9] In other words, when you eat adequate protein to keep you feeling full, you are less likely to overeat and consume excess calories from carbohydrates and fat to achieve that same feeling of fullness.

Another review of 37 research studies evaluated the effects of protein on body weight and found that people with high protein intake lost more weight compared to individuals consuming lower-protein diets of the same calorie level. Specifically, people who were prediabetic in these studies benefited the most from high-protein diets.[10]

A final study looked at the benefits of consuming more protein while trying to lose weight among older adults. It was found that those who had a higher protein intake on their weight loss diet were able to retain more lean body mass and lose more fat mass compared to those who had a lower protein intake.[11] This research highlights the importance of ensuring adequate protein intake for brain health — and weight loss.

WEIGHT LOSS ON THE MIND?

Research shows that higher-protein diets help with weight loss, body fat loss, reduction in inches around the waist, muscle maintenance, and improvement in blood pressure and triglycerides.

Higher-protein diets may be even more beneficial for people with prediabetes.

Older adults may be able to preserve more muscle and lose more fat when trying to lose weight on higher-protein diets.

Fish and poultry are higher-quality proteins that contain more protein per serving than plant sources of protein, such as beans and legumes. They contain the essential amino acids our bodies need, and these will be more readily absorbed and utilized by the body. This is why animal sources of protein are referred to as more "bioavailable," or "high biological value sources" of protein. Other high biological value sources include eggs, low-fat milk, and yogurt.

Of course, we are big fans of beans and legumes, which are an excellent source of proteins, especially for vegetarians and vegans. However, because most beans and legumes are not complete proteins and because they *also* contain carbohydrates, they have a different impact on blood sugar, satiety, and, in many cases, ultimate weight loss results. This is why I have chosen to group the beans and legumes with the carbohydrate foods, which we will discuss next.

CHAPTER 11

Carbohydrates: Whole Grains, Beans, and Legumes

The most important macronutrient for daily functioning is carbohydrates. Dietary carbohydrates (or carbs for short) provide 4 calories per gram; give foods flavor, texture, and moisture; and can also be added to foods (in the form of sugars) as preservatives to minimize bacterial growth and extend shelf life. Carbs get converted into sugar, or glucose, in the bloodstream. The glucose can be used for energy or stored in the muscles or liver for later use. Fiber, a nondigestible type of carb, helps maintain regular bowel function (insoluble fiber such as brown rice) and regulate cholesterol (soluble fiber such as oatmeal).

WHOLE GRAINS

Let's begin our discussion of the beneficial carbs with one of our most famous complex carb companions: whole grains (WG). In contrast to simple carbs such as highly processed grains—which are synonymous with sugars such as table sugar, honey, high-fructose corn syrup, and juices—complex carbs are digested and absorbed more slowly and are less likely to spike blood sugar.

We include whole grains in the MIND diet for a number of reasons. First, whole grains (as opposed to refined white grains like white rice, or bagels, bread, crackers, and other products made with white flour) have been demonstrated to lower the risk of developing heart disease and diabetes. Both of those chronic conditions are linked to greater risk of developing Alzheimer's, so whole grains are very important for a healthy diet. They are also a good source of vitamin E, folate, and B vitamins, which have been linked to good brain health and prevention of Alzheimer's. Research shows that the type of carbohydrate matters when it comes to risk for the aging brain. A review of research studies shows that diets high in complex carbohydrates were consistently found to be associated with improvements in short-term and long-term memory and cognition compared to diets high in refined carbohydrates and added sugars, which were shown to be associated with higher levels of Alzheimer's disease brain pathology markers.[1]

MIND DIET TARGET

Great Grains

Aim for 3 servings of whole grains per day.

1 serving = 1 slice bread or ½ cup cooked grains

Examples: 100% whole-grain breads, brown/wild rice, whole-grain pasta, quinoa, barley, bulgur, farro, whole-grain cereal, oats or oatmeal, whole-grain crackers

---

A whole grain is made up of three layers: the outer layer, or bran, which contains beneficial B vitamins and fiber; the white, starchy layer, or endosperm, which contains most of the calories in the form of carbohydrates; and a small seed as the inner layer, the germ or embryo, which is the most nutrient-dense component and carries the beneficial B vitamins, vitamin E, and unsaturated fats. When grains are "refined," the bran and germ are removed, leaving only the starchy endosperm, which strips the grain of its heart- and brain-healthy nutrients. Intake of whole grains is often recommended as a substitute for white, refined grains to help blood glucose levels become more stable from the high fiber content. Fiber helps the carbohydrate break down more slowly in the blood and gives the body more time to use the calories from this food source as energy, rather than store it as fat.

Be sure to always check the ingredient list to confirm if a product is whole grain. Unfortunately, product companies can be very misleading when it comes to advertising. The easiest way to identify if a product is whole grain is to look for the word "whole" in front of the grain listed as the first ingredient. Another quick check is to look for the 100% Whole Grain stamp on products. There are three different types of whole grain stamps on products, all with varying amounts of whole grain. The 100% stamp is the only one that ensures 100% of the product is made up of whole grains. The word "enriched" in the ingredient list would indicate that it is *not* a whole grain product. Enriched products have had nutrients *added back* to them after they were initially removed during processing. We recommend getting nutrients from foods in their natural, whole form as they will be best absorbed and used by the body.

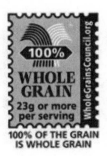

A study of almost 4,000 older adults found that those who met goals for whole grains as a part of the Mediterranean and DASH diets had significantly better cognitive functioning over a period of 11 years.[2] Researchers at Rush University Medical Center in Chicago continue to study the MIND diet in special populations and found that among Black Americans in particular, those who consumed more than 3 servings of whole grains per day (even higher than the MIND diet goal) had slower rates of cognitive decline in the areas of global cognition, perceptual speed, and episodic memory than those who consumed less than 1 serving daily.[3] The MIND diet goal is consistent with the 2020–2025 Dietary Guidelines for Americans recommendations to aim for 3 servings of whole grains daily to decrease risk for type 2 diabetes, high blood pressure, and high cholesterol.[4]

HOW TO ENJOY WHOLE GRAINS

Although 3 servings daily may seem like a lot, it's quite simple to meet the goal for whole grains each week. We will discuss more about appropriate food portions in part III, but it's common to have more than 1 serving of a MIND food in a single meal. For example, one slice of whole-grain bread is 1 serving of whole grains, but if you're eating a sandwich for lunch, you would be getting 2 servings in that portion of the meal. Likewise, ½ cup dry cereal or cooked oatmeal is 1 serving, but people often eat more than that, so a healthy portion would be 1 cup (2 servings) for breakfast.

In a Routine

Aim to start each day with 1 or 2 servings of whole grains. This MIND food is particularly beneficial in the morning, since the complex carbohydrates combined with the energizing B vitamins will provide a sustained source of energy to start your day off on the right track.

- **Choose the right bread.** Bread can be one of the trickiest products to identify as healthy while sifting through all the poor choices in the grocery store. Remember that the first step in identifying any whole-grain product is to look for "whole" leading the list of ingredients. Here are some other key things to look for when it comes to identifying healthy whole-grain breads:

○ *Fiber*: Breads should contain at least 3 grams of dietary fiber per slice.

○ *Sugar*: There should be no more than 2 grams of sugar per slice, and added sugars should be 0 grams.

○ *Total Carbohydrates*: Fiber and sugar *are* carbohydrates, which is why you find them indented underneath Total Carbohydrate on the food label. Look for breads with no more than 20 grams of total carbohydrate per slice. If you're trying to lose weight, you may want to seek out lower-carb breads, closer to 10 grams per slice. (We'll talk more about the role of carbohydrates and weight loss later.)

○ *Sodium*: Although some salt is needed for the preparation of bread, an excessive amount of sodium is often added as a flavor enhancer and to extend shelf life. A single slice of bread shouldn't contain more than 140 milligrams of sodium.

Here are some whole-grain bread brands I love, but I'll again remind you to please read the Nutrition Facts label for yourself, since products are forever changing! Dave's Killer Bread, Ezekiel 4:9 Sprouted Grain Bread, and Nature's Own 100% Whole Wheat Bread.

- **Go easy with avocado toast.** Smash an avocado, and mix with fresh lime juice, a pinch of cayenne pepper (optional), and a sprinkle of sea salt. Spread across whole-grain toast and enjoy! Add a hard-boiled or pan-fried egg to complete the meal with some quality protein.

- **Try other MIND toasts.** See part V for two more of Laura's creative ideas for morning toast options: Bonus Peanut Butter Toast (page 245) and Fancy Smoked Salmon Toast (page 246).

- **Mix up a grainy yogurt parfait.** Combine high-fiber cereal (at least 3 grams per serving) with low-fat Greek yogurt, and fresh or frozen berries, and top with crushed almonds (optional).

- **Make Hippie Oat Bowls (page 247).** I love Laura's MINDful take on traditional oatmeal in this recipe. This can be really simple to make with quick-cooking oatmeal and any nuts, seeds, and fruit available.

In a Rush

It's incredibly easy to meet your goal for whole grains when you are pressed for time. This is because most of them do not require refrigeration, special cleaning, or preparation before eating. If you have access only to packaged convenience items, the most important consideration is to make sure the product is 100 percent whole grain, as discussed above. My second piece of advice is to ensure that you pair a source of protein or unsaturated fat with your whole grain on the run, especially if you're going to be too busy to be paying close attention to your hunger cues. The protein will help the carb in the whole-grain food digest more slowly, allowing blood sugar levels to remain stable and prevent excessive hunger and overeating at your next meal.

Here are some "grab and go" meal or snack ideas:

- **Grab a whole-grain rice cake** (such as Lundberg brand) and top it:

  ○ Apple–peanut butter: Spread peanut (or other nut/seed) butter on a rice cake, top with apple slices, and sprinkle with ground cinnamon and fresh lemon juice (optional).

  ○ Greek-style: Spread hummus on a rice cake, top with 1 slice reduced-fat cheese, cucumber and tomato slices, and fresh lemon juice, and sprinkle with a pinch of sea salt and fresh or dried dill (optional).

- **Try whole-grain crackers**, such as Wasa Crispbread, Triscuit Original (the original product should list just three ingredients: whole-grain wheat, canola oil, and sea salt), or Trader Joe's Norwegian Crispbread, paired with the following:

  - A schmear of nut butter or hummus

  - Tuna or chicken salad

  - Sliced avocado and tomato

  - A hard-boiled egg

  - Low-fat cheese

- **Snack MINDfully.** Technically, snack foods such as the crackers listed above, some pretzels (remember to check the ingredient list for the word "whole"), and popcorn are whole grains. However, it's important to be familiar with your patterns around certain foods. I've had many people tell me, and I've experienced for myself, that it can be difficult to control intake of certain snack foods like crackers, popcorn, and pretzels—even the whole-grain kind! If you know that snack foods like these are a trigger for you to overeat, I'd recommend choosing other foods. Additionally, you should be MINDful about what you're eating *with* these snack foods if you do choose them. For example, pairing full-fat cheese with whole-grain crackers or melting a stick of butter and piling mounds of salt on top of popcorn will likely negate the beneficial effects of the whole grains. Some healthier alternatives include pairing a low-fat cheese with whole-grain crackers or trading the butter on fresh-popped popcorn for a drizzle of EVOO and even a sprinkle of fresh or dried herbs such as dill or rosemary—or check out the health food aisle for nutritional yeast as a vegan substitute for cheese. (See Laura's recipe for Olive Oil Popcorn on page 301.)

THE BAD RAP FOR WHOLE GRAINS: SETTLING THE SCORE

There have been a few fad diet books that claim that whole grains contribute to inflammation in the body. Yet it is important to base recommendations on data rather than on theory. Both the Mediterranean and DASH diets (which have been rigorously tested with randomized intervention trials) recommend many servings of whole grains per day. These trials have all looked at markers of inflammation in the body, and the science is clear that the people with high whole grains in their diets have lower levels of inflammation. For people who suffer from gluten intolerance or sensitivities, we recommend they choose whole grains that don't have gluten in them, such as quinoa, amaranth, gluten-free oats, millet, and brown rice.

BEANS AND LEGUMES

Beans and legumes (Bn) share many heart- and brain-healthy nutrients with whole grains, including B vitamins such as folate and B_6, enabling new DNA to be built, protecting cells against oxidative injury, and keeping inflammation controlled. The previously mentioned report looking at data from the Nurses' Health Study and protein's effect on subjective cognitive decline found that beans and legumes were associated with a 28 percent lower risk for cognitive decline for every 3 additional weekly servings.[5] The MIND diet's recommendation to get 3 servings of beans and legumes each week is consistent with the 2020–2025 Dietary Guidelines for Americans recommendations for these foods to promote cardioprotective benefits.[6]

MIND DIET TARGET

Beans for the Brain

Consume 3 servings of beans and legumes each week.

1 serving = ½ cup canned or cooked

Examples: black, pinto, cannellini, kidney, lima, red/white, and navy beans; chickpeas; lentils; tofu; soybeans (edamame); hummus

HOW TO ENJOY BEANS AND LEGUMES

Beans and legumes provide a vegetarian source of protein, although most of them are not complete proteins. The exact composition varies depending on the type of bean/legume, but for most, about one-third of the macronutrient composition comes from protein and about two-thirds from carbohydrates, with less than 5 percent coming from fat. That is why I have grouped them in the carbohydrates chapter. They are, however, complex carbohydrates that are high in fiber and excellent for inducing satiety, and they can be a great component of a weight loss plan if you are MINDful of portion size and overall carbohydrate intake.

In a Routine

- **Add beans to your weekly salad.** I'm going to refer to my refrigerator filled with storage containers of salad ingredients once again, because it's just so easy to get into a routine of eating weekly salads *without* getting bored by keeping these items handy and changing up the ingredients each week. Let's add beans and legumes to the container count. I rotate canned chickpeas, cannellini beans, and kidney beans regularly. If you're using canned items, remember to purchase low-sodium and rinse thoroughly, especially if you have high blood pressure.

- **Use beans as filler.** Get into the habit of using beans and legumes as a hearty filler for soups, stews, and casseroles. You might also consider getting your fill with a three-bean salad of kidney beans, black beans, and chickpeas mixed with red onions and an EVOO–balsamic vinegar dressing. Add your favorite herbs, such as dried oregano, parsley, basil, rosemary, or Italian blend. You could even throw in a fourth "bean"—green beans—to add a serving of other vegetables and make this salad a heart-healthy side dish. For other creative ways to incorporate beans and legumes into routine dishes, see Laura's recipes for Chickpea Tuna Salad (page 273) and Black Bean Veggie Burgers (page 277).

- **Whip up some homemade hummus.** This is one of my favorite dishes to make at home instead of buying the store-bought version, because I can choose the seasonings and other ingredients myself to control the intensity of the flavors and nutritional value. I find a lot of store-bought hummus options to be too garlicky and not as fresh tasting as my homemade version. You don't need a fancy food processor to make this; you can really use any blender. I use my portable NutriBullet to blend canned chickpeas, fresh garlic (just ½ clove for me!), tahini (or any nut/seed butter if I don't have tahini on hand), and lemon juice. I simply keep adding, blending, and tasting until it reaches the consistency and flavor that I'm happy with. For a unique and delicious hummus using black beans, check out Laura's recipe for Spicy Black Bean Hummus (page 300).

- **Make MINDful bean swaps.** Here are some easy suggestions to substitute beans and legumes for typical meal ingredients:

  - Smashed lentils or chickpeas instead of ground meat for meatballs

  - Hummus or black bean spread instead of cream cheese or butter on a bagel or toast

- Smashed black or kidney beans instead of tomato sauce on a cauliflower crust, topped with low-fat cheese for a bean and veggie pizza

In a Rush

- **Grab a complete protein quickie.** Edamame (Japanese soybeans that have been boiled or steamed) and lupini beans (native to the Mediterranean) contain all nine essential amino acids that the body cannot produce on its own, making these MIND foods complete proteins. Although these options still contain some carbohydrates, they also contain a higher concentration of protein, and you may find them to be even more satisfying in smaller portions. This makes them a great option for a complete snack, since they are higher in protein than other beans and legumes but are still a quality, high-fiber source of complex carbohydrates to keep blood sugar stable and energy levels sustained until your next meal or snack. Both of these beans can be eaten hot, but I love them cold with a splash of low-sodium soy sauce or liquid aminos if you're looking for an even lower-sodium substitute.

- **Dip into some hummus or black bean dip.** Whether store-bought or homemade, these dips are easy to pair with raw veggies such as baby carrots, cucumber slices, bell pepper strips, celery stalks, or whole-grain pretzels, crackers, or rice cakes.

- **Go roasted for chickpeas.** Many grocery stores carry various flavors of roasted chickpeas for a satisfying snack. Two popular brands are the Good Bean and Saffron Road. Remember to check the sodium content and aim for snacks at or below 300 milligrams if you have high blood pressure. You can also make these easily at home by draining and rinsing a can of chickpeas, patting them dry, and tossing them with your favorite herbs and spices and a touch of EVOO on a rimmed baking sheet. Roast at 400°F for 20 to 30 minutes or to the desired crispness.

- **Grab a frozen burrito.** For me, this one goes in the "In a Rush" *and* in the "In a Routine" section. I am guilty of being "too busy" at least once a week to prepare a balanced meal on a workday. To guard against making impulsive decisions that lead to poor food choices, I try to choose among a select few items that provide good nutrition without excess saturated fat and preservatives. My favorite way to get in a serving of beans throughout the week is with an Amy's Organic bean and cheese burrito. The saturated fat falls under 3 grams, it provides a full serving of beans, and it's wrapped in a whole-grain tortilla. I pair this with at least 2 servings of salad from a bagged fresh salad kit. As always with packaged products, keep an eye on sodium levels and aim for meal totals around 600 milligrams or less if you have high blood pressure.

CARBOHYDRATES AND WEIGHT LOSS

A meta-analysis of studies that included more than 6,000 adults concluded that low-carbohydrate diets were superior to low-fat diets when it comes to weight loss, reduction of triglycerides, and boosting HDL cholesterol.[7] One interesting finding was that the low-carbohydrate diets did not fare better in terms of LDL cholesterol and total cholesterol, suggesting that more than just overall macronutrient intake must be taken into consideration when making food choices. According to this study, the type of carbohydrates (and fats) we choose to eat really does matter when it comes to heart health. This is consistent with what we have discussed earlier in terms of whole-grain carbs over their white, refined counterparts and choosing unsaturated fats over saturated fats for prevention of cognitive decline.

The MIND diet counts beans and whole grains as carbs. Technically, all fruits, including berries, also contain carbohydrates. But as discussed earlier, compared to all other fruits, berries are the lowest in sugar and highest in fiber, and have been the only fruit shown to be protective against cognitive decline; therefore, we will keep our berry friends grouped with the leafy greens and other veggies.

Carbohydrates	MIND Food Points	
Whole Grains (WG) **Goal:** 3 servings/day **Serving size:** 1 slice bread or ½ cup cooked grains	0–4 servings/week	0
	5–20 servings/week	0.5
	21+ servings/week	1
Beans & Legumes (Bn) **Goal:** 3 servings/week **Serving size:** ½ cup canned or cooked	0 servings/week	0
	1–2 servings/week	0.5
	3+ servings/week	1

Both fiber and sugar are carbohydrates. Fiber is much more nutritious and, as discussed, acts to keep our gut healthy and ensure regular bowel movements and regulate cholesterol levels in the blood. Sugars are needed as the first source of fuel for activity, but most Americans get too much sugar in their diet. The foods that count as carbs on the MIND diet *Foods to Limit* list are fried foods and sweets and pastries. For most of us, it's not difficult to eat—or overeat—carbs. Most foods that are readily available at restaurants, cafés, convenience stores, vending machines, or even right in our home pantries are carbs.

Let's dive a little deeper into how choosing quality carbohydrates could impact weight loss. For example, 1 cup of cooked 100 percent whole-grain brown rice and 1 cup of white rice have the same amount of calories and carbohydrates, so it might be easy to assume that they are equivalent in terms of their effects on weight loss. However, without the fiber and other beneficial nutrients provided from the whole grains within the brown rice, the white rice may not make you feel full after eating only 1 cup and you may end up eating a lot more. This is common with many white, starchy carb products. When was the last time you portioned out (or even noticed) the suggested serving size of white pasta, a bowl of starchy cereal, a fried food like french fries or potato chips (yep, potato chips count as fried foods!), or sweets and pastries such as ice cream (a serving of ice cream is ½ cup, by the way)? In other words, it will likely be difficult for you to "stick to" a small portion of carbohydrate without the adequate fiber and nutrients that whole grains and/or protein provide. The bottom line: it's all about balance.

Remember, the goal of the MIND diet is not to be perfect 100 percent of the time. If you end up choosing the white pasta, eat more cereal than the serving on the box suggests, indulge in fried foods on occasion, or eat more than ½ cup of ice cream, that doesn't mean your entire eating pattern is doomed. This is why it's so useful to keep up with the weekly tracking of your MIND foods, which we explain how to do in part III. That way, you can plan for (or at least be aware of) indulgences and make more MINDful choices to balance the score for the week.

For weight loss, many people benefit from reducing the amount of carbs eaten (especially from white, refined grains, fried foods, sweets and pastries, and sweet drinks) and increasing intake of vegetables and berries. As discussed in chapter 10, protein is also a crucial component in a complete, satisfying meal. We will talk more about how to design balanced MIND meals in part III.

WEIGHT LOSS ON THE MIND?

For the best weight loss results, balance small portions of high-fiber, quality carbs from whole grains and/or beans with leafy greens and other vegetables and quality proteins from fish or poultry.

CHAPTER 12

Wine in Moderation

The literature on alcohol consumption and dementia is fairly consistent. People who consume very moderate levels—anywhere from 1 to 7 drinks per week for women and no more than 14 drinks per week for men—have the lowest risk of dementia. However, every drink that you consume above those very moderate levels actually contributes to brain atrophy, since alcohol is harmful to neurons. For some reason, a very moderate intake appears to be healthy for the brain.

First, let's define what is meant by the word "moderation." It's a term that is unfortunately overused, especially when it comes to health and wellness. Moderation is often defined as the balance between extremes or an avoidance of excesses in one's actions, beliefs, or behaviors. In my experience, people have often used "moderation" as a way to justify poor eating behaviors.

My approach is to encourage people to embrace moderation as an opportunity to be flexible and not feel tied to a specific set of rules. Moderation can afford you the freedom to choose when you want to safely indulge in various actions, as long as you are paying attention to when those actions become repeated behaviors that transform into unhealthy habits. With diet and nutrition, I specifically encourage people to pay attention to how various foods make the body feel—both positively and negatively. With this type of attention over time, you'll likely discover that the urge to make unhealthy choices diminishes as you begin to appreciate the benefits you reap from healthy food choices.

The only item in the moderation category on the list of MIND diet 10 *Foods to Choose* list is wine (Win).

MIND DIET TARGET

Wine Not?

Consume wine in moderation—up to 1 serving per day.

1 serving = 5 fluid ounces

Examples: red wine, white wine, sparkling wine

Wine consumption has long been a topic under investigation for health benefits due to its beneficial nutrients, including polyphenols such as anthocyanins, and resveratrol, which is more concentrated in red wine. You may recall that these are also brain-healthy nutrients common to berries. A review of studies exploring the relationship between wine consumption and cognition and dementia concluded that light to moderate wine consumption has been demonstrated to be protective for the brain, while excessive consumption has been shown to be harmful.[1] In addition to these nutrients' antioxidant and anti-inflammatory properties, other suggested mechanisms may be the ability of resveratrol to prevent beta-amyloid protein buildup in the brain; but studies have shown that in order for resveratrol to provide this benefit, excessive amounts of wine would need to be consumed, which is certainly not recommended.[2]

Research on the connection between alcohol and cognitive decline was evaluated in a review of studies, underscoring that light to moderate alcohol consumption may protect against dementia and Alzheimer's disease; however, due to lack of evidence on the risks of increasing alcohol consumption for nondrinkers, the current suggestion is for nondrinkers to continue to abstain.[3]

Research on how much alcohol to drink is consistent with MIND diet recommendations—as shown in the MIND food points section for wine, anywhere from 1 to 7 drinks in a week will score you 0.5 or 1 point, but consumption above 1 drink per day (more than 7 drinks in a week) *or* having no drinks puts your MIND food points for wine at 0 points for the week. Wine consumption has also been shown to be protective to the heart by boosting HDL cholesterol and improving blood flow. And we know that what is healthy for the heart is also healthy for the brain!

Moderation		MIND Food Points	
Wine (Win) **Goal:** 1 serving/day **Serving size:** 5 fluid ounces		0 servings/week	0
		1–6 servings/week	0.5
		7 servings/week	1
		8+ servings/week	0.5

But remember, if you are not a current drinker or are not used to drinking wine at this frequency, please don't increase your intake. We know that alcohol is addictive and can interfere with logical reasoning and thinking, lowering inhibitions and increasing the likelihood of engaging in other risky behaviors (such as overeating). It's best to avoid an increase in overall alcohol consumption, especially if you're trying to lose weight. Alcohol is technically the fourth macronutrient, providing 7 calories per gram—almost double that of protein or carbohydrates.

I often work with people who struggle to understand why they are having trouble losing weight, and alcohol consumption is a common reason. It can be easy to forget about beverage intake when you are not paying attention or when your judgment becomes impaired. This can be especially important for individuals with existing health complications like obesity or type 2 diabetes. In the Look AHEAD study, more than 5,000 participants were put either into an intensive lifestyle intervention that included goals for physical activity and nutrition and restricted alcohol intake to 1 or 2 drinks per day or into a diabetes support and education group.[4] Those who participated in the intensive lifestyle group and abstained from drinking alcohol lost more weight compared to those who drank alcohol. Furthermore, the participants who drank alcohol had a more difficult time keeping their weight off. This shows the negative impact that alcohol can make, despite efforts to eat healthy and exercise, especially for those who are already obese or have diabetes.

Here's something you can try if you want to find out for sure if alcohol is keeping you from reaching your goal: keep everything the same for at least 4 weeks, except for the alcohol. Remove all alcohol for this short period of time as an experiment. If you begin to see the needle move...there's your answer. Does that mean that you must give up alcohol completely? Perhaps not, but it's likely that you will learn a lot about yourself in the process, which could give you insight into what might be getting in the way. If you're not quite ready to kick the habit just yet, another option would be to carefully keep a journal just of alcohol intake for 4 weeks. Narrowing the focus to one area can help bring awareness to potential problems.

WEIGHT LOSS ON THE MIND?

Drinking alcohol may impair your ability to lose and maintain your weight, especially if you are obese or have type 2 diabetes.

Boozy Experiment:

Option 1: Cut out all alcohol for 4 weeks. Observe results. Proceed as desired.

Option 2: Keep a detailed log of all alcohol consumed for 4 weeks. Observe frequency and volume. Adjust as needed.

Just as with all other aspects of the MIND diet, you're in control when it comes to the decision of how much alcohol you'll consume, if any. My job is to ensure that you are informed of the benefits and risks, and that you feel fully empowered to be able to answer the question, "Wine not?"

CHAPTER 13

Saturated Fats: Red Meat, Butter, Cheese, Fried Foods, and Sweets

The key distinguishing characteristic between the *Foods to Choose* and *Foods to Limit* is the concentration of saturated fat. Diets high in saturated and trans fats have been shown to increase the risk for cardiovascular disease, insulin resistance, type 2 diabetes, cancer, and systemic inflammation.[1] Dr. Morris and her research group were studying the effects of dietary fats on Alzheimer's disease long before they developed the MIND diet. After following a cohort of more than 800 older adults for up to 4 years, those who had the highest intakes of saturated fat had the fastest rates of cognitive decline and twice the risk of developing Alzheimer's disease compared to those who had the lowest intakes of saturated fat.[2] Current dietary guidelines for Americans recommend no more than 10 percent of daily calories from saturated fat.[3]

Much controversy has been generated over the years regarding dietary fat consumption. The low-fat diet craze in the 1980s and '90s caused people to drastically reduce total overall fat intake, with an unfortunate increase in overall carbohydrate and refined sugar intake. Then emerged evidence of refined carbohydrate diets causing obesity and cardiovascular complications, followed by the low-carb diet craze during the early part of the new millennium, with people celebrating by trading their bowl of oatmeal for a morning plate of steak and eggs with a side of bacon and a cup of coffee with a dollop of butter. Women from the Nurses' Health Study and men from the Health Professionals Follow-Up Study were evaluated over roughly a 30-year period spanning the age of the diet craze to determine if the specific type of fat they consumed was associated with cause of death.[4] Higher intakes of saturated fat and trans fat were associated with higher rates of death. In contrast, higher intakes of mono- and polyunsaturated fats were associated with lower death rates. As it turns out, butter really *isn't* better!

Instead of eliminating an entire food group, the recommendation is to replace foods high in saturated fat (red meat, butter, full-fat cheese, fried foods, sweets and pastries) with those rich in mono- and polyunsaturated fats (EVOO, nuts, and fatty fish). This does not mean that you need to eliminate all foods that contain saturated fat. Remember that it is a *limit* list, not an *avoid* list. The targets were carefully designed to match what the research shows in terms of ideal intakes to slow cognitive decline combined with the most evidence-based national health guidelines.

MIND DIET TARGETS

Replace Saturated Fats with Mono- and Polyunsaturated Fats

Consume less red meat, butter, full-fat cheese, fried foods, and sweets and pastries.

Replace with EVOO, nuts, and fatty fish.

I've never been the type of coach that likes to tell people only what *not* to do, which is why I have continued to emphasize the idea of moderation and fully owning and enjoying whatever choices you make. But here are some ideas for healthier substitutes for when you are trying to reduce the foods on the list to limit:

- **"Meat" your limit.** Red meat and processed meats such as bacon, sausage, hot dogs, bologna, salami, and other cold cuts are rich in saturated fat, sodium, and calories. A 1-ounce serving of red meat has about 100 calories, making a 4-ounce serving (about the size of a woman's palm) a whopping 400 calories. A good polyunsaturated option would be salmon or albacore tuna for a dose of omega-3s. Even if you're not in it for the omegas, it would still be beneficial to sub any other fish or switch up the protein to skinless, white-meat turkey or chicken or even a vegetarian source such as tofu. **Limit red meats and processed meats to no more than 3 servings per week.**

- **Butter...it's not really better.** Butter and stick margarine contain not only saturated fats, but often trans fats as well. As mentioned previously, trans fats are particularly harmful since they raise harmful LDL cholesterol and decrease protective HDL cholesterol. These products are also typically high in sodium. A nice substitute for butter to provide monounsaturated fatty acids is EVOO, which can be used to replace it in almost any recipe or dish. In baking, if a recipe calls for butter or stick margarine/shortening, you can simply replace 50 percent with a fruit puree such as applesauce. For example, if a recipe calls for 1 cup (2 sticks) butter, a reasonable replacement would be to use ½ cup (1 stick) butter + ½ cup applesauce. Lastly, many commercial products now exist that are more responsibly produced and do not create trans fats in the processing. I recommend Earth Balance or Smart Balance Omega blend. Please always remember to check your nutrition labels, since new products are being distributed every day! Aim for no more than 3 grams of saturated fat per serving and always look for products with 0 grams of trans fat. **Limit butter and stick margarine to 1 teaspoon or less each day.**

- **Cheese...please?** In the United States, one of the biggest contributors to saturated fat is full-fat cheese, which is also high in sodium and is calorie-dense. A 1-ounce serving of full-fat cheese (about the size of four dice or two dominos) has around 100 calories. It can be easy to forget that cheese is often paired with other food items that seem to be a natural part of some popular foods, such as pizza, macaroni and cheese, cheeseburgers, etc. One strategy for this group is to choose light or reduced-fat cheese for quick snacks such as part-skim mozzarella string cheese (a fan favorite among the kiddos!), reduced-fat provolone on turkey wraps and sandwiches, and low-fat ricotta cheese in recipes with other bold flavors, and then save the "real" cheese indulgences for when you can fully appreciate it, such as when you're out with friends and everyone is sharing pizza or when you're pairing a good cheese with a nice glass of wine if that's something you enjoy. It's all about choices. **Limit full-fat cheese to 2 ounces or less each week.**

- **Don't get fried out.** This one feels like it needs no explanation of reasons to limit, since fried foods are loaded with saturated fat, sodium, and calories. My recommendation here is to be on the lookout for items that are being masked as healthy but have all the components of being fried out. For example, it may be easy to overlook that snack foods such as potato and tortilla chips are indeed fried. Additionally, many varieties of frozen chicken tenders or nuggets and french fries or tater tots may have instructions to bake in the oven but have originally been fried before they were frozen. One of my favorite inventions has been the air fryer, which works by circulating air at high pressure and temperature, requiring minimal oil to produce a crisp product with even less cleanup than deep-frying. I highly recommend this as an investment if possible. **Limit fried foods to no more than 1 serving weekly.**

- **Life is sweet.** As mentioned, sweets, pastries, and sweet drinks pop up on the list of MIND diet *Foods to Limit* because of both saturated and trans fat content and added sugars. Saturated fats and added sugars have been linked to obesity, high cholesterol, and diabetes. These are all independent risk factors for development of cognitive decline and dementia, so being MINDful of intake for both fats and sugars is crucial to a heart- and brain-healthy dietary pattern. This is why the category of sweets and pastries also includes sugar-sweetened beverages such as regular sodas, sports drinks, energy drinks, sweetened waters, coffees, and teas. Healthy substitutes for sweets can include fresh or frozen berries or savoring an ounce or two of dark chocolate. If you're looking to get in some mono- and polyunsaturated fats, try almonds, walnuts, a mixture of herb-roasted nuts or seeds, and/or some green or black olives as an after-dinner treat. Alternatively, you may decide to choose your daily glass of wine as your dessert. Again, life is about choices, and they are meant to be savored and enjoyed. **Limit sweets and pastries to 4 or fewer servings each week.**

See the following table for a summary of ideas for ways to swap out saturated and trans fats for healthier unsaturated fats or other MIND foods.

FAT SWAPS	
Instead of Saturated and Trans Fats	**Choose Mono- and Polyunsaturated Fats**
Red and processed meats such as bacon, sausage, hot dogs, bologna, salami, and other cold cuts	Non-fried fish and seafood, such as salmon, albacore tuna, or sardines
Butter and stick margarine, coconut oil, palm oil	Extra-virgin, avocado, grapeseed, sesame, or canola oils, or heart-healthy spread
Full-fat cheese, including on pizza and burgers/sandwiches, cream cheese, etc.	Reduced-fat cheese, nutritional yeast, nuts and nut butters, seeds such as chia or flax, or soybeans/edamame
Fried foods, including any deep-fried meats or fish, french fries, potato chips, tortilla chips, etc.	Baked meats, poultry, or seafood, oven-fried or air-fried potatoes, kale chips, beet chips, etc.
Sweets, pastries, and processed foods made with partially hydrogenated oils	Berries, nuts and nut butters, seeds such as chia or flax, avocados, olives, wine in moderation

BONUS: SUGAR SWAPS	
Regular sodas, sports drinks, energy drinks, and sweetened waters, coffees, and teas	Water, plain or sweetened with berries and lime/lemon juice, seltzer waters, unsweetened iced or hot teas

Saturated Fats	MIND Food Points	
Red & Processed Meats (RM) **Goal:** 0–3 servings/week **Serving size:** 3–5 ounces	0–3 servings/week	1
	4–6 servings/week	0.5
	7+ servings/week	0
Butter & Stick Margarine (But) **Goal:** 0–1 serving/day **Serving size:** 1 teaspoon	0–7 servings/week	1
	8–13 servings/week	0.5
	14+ servings/week	0
Full-Fat Cheese (Chs) **Goal:** 0–2 servings/week **Serving size:** 1 ounce	0–2 servings/week	1
	3–6 servings/week	0.5
	7+ servings/week	0
Fried Foods (Fri) **Goal:** 0–1 serving/week **Serving size:** 1 serving	0–1 serving/week	1
	2–3 servings/week	0.5
	4+ servings/week	0
Sweets, Pastries & Sweet Drinks (Swt) **Goal:** 0–4 servings/week **Serving size:** 1 treat or 8-ounce drink	0–4 servings/week	1
	5–6 servings/week	0.5
	7+ servings/week	0

COOKING METHODS MATTER: ADVANCED GLYCATION END PRODUCTS

Awareness about the foods we eat, as well as the cooking methods we use, is important to brain health and longevity. This is especially true for the *Foods to Limit*. Advanced glycation end products (AGEs) are compounds that can be produced naturally in the body, causing inflammation and oxidative stress, and have been linked to acceleration of cognitive decline. Although AGEs have typically been shown to be higher in people with diabetes and kidney disease, they can also build up in healthy people who consume foods that have high levels of sugar combined with high levels of animal protein cooked at high heat (think barbecue sauce on ribs, a chocolate-glazed doughnut, or classic french fries).

A study of almost 700 older adults from the MAP cohort evaluated the impact of AGEs from red meat, high-sugar packaged and processed foods, full-fat cheese, poultry, and fish based on the cooking method used to prepare these foods (frying, grilling, boiling, roasting, etc.).[5] It was found that higher AGE levels in the body were associated with faster cognitive decline. In fact, those individuals who had the highest levels had a 50 percent faster rate of decline in cognition compared to those who had the lowest levels. Furthermore, the researchers determined that this was true even for individuals who had no diabetes or other cardiovascular disease risk factors, suggesting that these harmful compounds could be present and causing long-term damage to the brain even in healthy people.

The good news is that this is another component you can control! In addition to monitoring your intake of AGEs through the MIND diet targets for the *Foods to Limit*, you can also reduce the probability of AGE building up as you age by more often choosing lower-heat cooking methods for animal proteins, such as poaching and steaming, versus high-heat grilling and frying. When you do cook with high heat, consider marinating proteins in a mixture that contains citrus such as lemon or lime juice or a vinegar base for about an hour. The acid can reduce the AGEs produced. As always, remember to balance your meal with plenty of the plant-based foods naturally low in AGEs, such as veggies, berries, whole grains, and beans.

CHAPTER 14

MIND Diet FAQs:
Lessons Learned from the Field

There are so many things we have learned along the way from many of our research studies over the years that make the MIND diet what it is today. We were able to continue to refine the targets of each individual food to be tailored to match eating habits that were more conducive to practical behaviors. We were also able to better understand where the diet needed to be tailored for individual food preferences, cultural habits, dietary restrictions, and even food allergies. As a result, we compiled a list of frequently asked questions (FAQs) that was inspired by real questions from real people "in the field."

Dairy and eggs: Do I need to be concerned about cholesterol?

Dairy products, such as milk and yogurt, have not been shown to influence brain health but can be a part of a healthy diet. The MIND diet recommends reducing full-fat cheese and butter or stick margarines due to the high amount of saturated fat. Eggs are a great source of protein and brain-healthy nutrients such as vitamins D and B_{12}. The American Heart Association states that up to 1 egg yolk every day is safe if you do not have existing cardiovascular disease. Remember, dietary cholesterol does not increase cholesterol levels; rather, saturated fat does. When consuming dairy products, it is best to choose low-fat versions, such as nonfat or low-fat milk and yogurt.

Why aren't other fruits on the MIND diet?

As discussed previously, research shows that berries have a protective effect on the brain above and beyond other types of fruits. Additionally, berries are the lowest in sugar and highest in fiber and therefore the best fruit to eat for healthy weight management. Other fruit is not discouraged, but also not recommended in unlimited amounts, since fruit contains natural sugars that will raise blood sugar. A diet rich in both fruits and vegetables has shown to be involved in reducing risk for diabetes, high blood pressure, obesity, and high cholesterol, all of which are modifiable risk factors for Alzheimer's disease.

Do cherries count as berries?

Cherries are a stone fruit (not a berry) and belong to the *Prunus* family. While cherries do contain polyphenol flavonoids that can act as antioxidants to clear free radicals and prevent inflammation, they are not included in the MIND diet. This is because cherries specifically have not been studied extensively enough to ensure that they can have an impact on cognitive decline. As stated throughout this book, we are presenting to you only the most researched evidence to ensure you have the most powerful tools for your brain-healthy eating pattern.

Why are sugar-sweetened beverages, such as regular soda, fruit juice and drinks, sport and energy drinks, sweetened waters, and coffee and tea beverages with added sugars, included with the sweets and pastries on the Foods to Limit *list if these drinks do not contain saturated fat?*

Sugar-sweetened beverages were originally *not* counted as foods to limit when the MIND diet was first created.[1] Since that time, our research team has revised this and other categories to match the most recent evidence on foods that may be harmful to the brain. The MIND diet emphasizes that the common nutritional thread on the list of *Foods to Limit* is saturated fat, but sugar-sweetened beverages have more recently been added to the list because, as with sweets and pastries, research shows that they are associated with heart disease, diabetes, and obesity—all secondary risk factors for cognitive decline.[2]

Do I need to monitor my sodium intake?

Although making a conscious effort to keep sodium intake low was a prime feature of the DASH diet, tracking sodium is not a focus of the MIND diet. This is due to the repeatedly mentioned concept that being MINDful of portions and frequency of the food categories on the MIND diet's lists of *Foods to Choose* and *Foods to Limit* should allow you to consume other foods in moderation and therefore fall within a healthful range for other unhealthy nutrients such as sodium. All of the foods on the list of *Foods to Choose* are naturally low in sodium, and most of those on the list of *Foods to Limit* are quite high, which should allow for a balance of the nutrients when following the diet at least moderately well. In part III we will talk about specific targets for those interested in watching sodium levels.

What about coconut oil?

The research to date is not supportive of intake of coconut oil and related products for memory preservation. We recommend using EVOO first; a small amount of coconut oil for flavor is acceptable. Coconut oil is high in saturated fat, which we know is connected to increased risk for heart disease, stroke, and cognitive decline.

Should I take a multivitamin supplement?

Similar to the omega-3 fatty acid supplementation discussion in the fish chapter, the consensus in the field of experts for brain health and cognition is that a multivitamin supplement is not currently recommended based on the available evidence.[3] One well-designed study by Dr. Laura Baker, leader of the U.S. POINTER trial, investigated a standardized multivitamin and mineral supplement against a supplement containing high levels of cocoa extract rich in flavanols.[4] The cocoa extract did not show a beneficial effect on cognition, but the multivitamin and mineral supplement alone showed promising effects, improving cognition in the areas of memory and executive function, which suggests the potential for this type of supplement to improve cognition in older adults. The authors assert that further investigation is needed to replicate the results before clinical recommendations can be made. Multivitamin and mineral supplements should not be a substitute for a healthy diet and overall lifestyle changes. More research is needed before supplementation of any kind will be adopted into public health recommendations for brain health in the absence of deficiency.

PART III

YOUR MIND DIET TOOLBOX FOR SUCCESS

"If you want to become better at something, research it. Increase your understanding, ask questions, and learn all you can about it. The more tools and knowledge you collect to help you toward your goals, the more likely you are to succeed."

—*Dr. Martha Clare Morris*

CHAPTER 15

The Essential Tools

By Jennifer Ventrelle

Before we jump into the 6-week program, it is imperative that you have a good understanding of all the tools you will need to succeed. Here, we will go over key strategies that have shown to be successful in implementing behavior changes and aiding in weight loss. We would like you to be able to use these approaches time and time again for long-term success. The idea is for you to curate habits that fit your own unique routine and help you live the life you want.

> "As a type 2 diabetic, I have tried for years to eat wisely, but the concise manner in which the MIND diet introduces strong, research-based nutritional guidelines and the extraordinarily well-designed method for assessing diet quality have impressed me powerfully."
>
> —*Abigail B.*

Let's get started on learning the tools you will use to have the best experience possible throughout the 6-week program—and beyond! The people who have been the most successful in following the MIND diet (that is, those who achieved MIND diet scores at or above 12.5, the high end of the range shown to be most protective for the brain) *and* have been able to maintain or achieve healthy weight goals have a few things in common. We have summarized these practices into the five "SMART MIND" habits for success:

1. Self-Monitoring

2. Meal Planning

3. Action Planning

4. Reflection

5. Trust and Support

In this section, we'll introduce you to each of the habits and invite you to gather the tools that will help you along the way. We will also guide you on how to use the tools so that you're prepared to begin the 6-week program in chapter 18. A key thing to remember as you explore the guidelines and suggested tools is that we will present a variety of options for you to choose what works best for you. The program is meant to be one that can be integrated within an existing lifestyle—even if you're already motivated to follow a special diet for health, cultural, environmental, or any other reasons.

Research supports the idea that a variety of healthy eating patterns can be modified to fit individual preferences and that a Mediterranean-type diet such as the MIND diet may be superior when it comes to cardiovascular protection and prevention of cognitive decline.[1] The message is that you should feel free to *simultaneously* follow any other special dietary guideline while going through this program. Vegetarians and vegans can find plenty of plant-based recipes to get a therapeutic MIND score, low-carb eaters could reduce the whole-grain target and focus on other non-carbohydrate MIND foods to boost their score, and intermittent fasters could certainly feast on a variety of MIND foods during their eating window and on nonfasting days. The goal here is a customized toolbox available for you to build your own path to success. Here is a snapshot of all the tools you'll need for a successful 6-week program:

SMART MIND TOOLBOX FOR SUCCESS

Tool #1: MIND Diet Refrigerator Chart
Tool #2: Calendar with Reminders
Tool #3: Menu Plan and Recipe Bank
Tool #4: Grocery Shopping and Meal Preparation Plan
Tool #5: MIND Plate for Meal Planning
Tool #6: Small Goals List
Tool #7: Reflection and Gratitude Journal
Tool #8: Social Support Partner

You will learn that the basic structure for the 6 weeks will be the same, allowing you to set the foundation for ongoing weekly habits, rather than a "diet" that lasts only a few weeks and may leave you feeling depleted. At the end of this program, we want you to feel empowered with the right tools and to have curated routines and habits to live your best life.

SELF-MONITORING

Self-monitoring is listed as the first SMART MIND habit for a reason! This is one of the most effective ways to implement change in any behavior. It is a way of having accountability. There are many feelings that can come up with this practice: it can be a huge responsibility and extremely freeing at the same time. Ultimately, you may find that keeping yourself accountable will improve the relationship you have with yourself and those around you. In the early phases of learning something new, the ability to monitor, evaluate, and correct yourself is vital. Think of a young child learning to walk. If you ran over to pick her up and console her each time she fell, without letting her learn how to get up on her own, she might attach a negative association to the experience of walking, which could delay her ability to become independent with this crucial life skill. In research involving 20,000 people across 26 studies, participants were asked to change their eating behaviors by monitoring intake and receiving automated feedback via computerized reports with no help from a health provider or coach. It was found that those who self-monitored what they consumed made significant dietary changes compared to those who did not monitor their intake, highlighting the power of tracking eating habits.[2]

The MIND Diet Refrigerator Chart is your self-monitoring savior here and is the first tool (and perhaps one of the most critical) to assist you in the program.

Tool #1: The MIND Diet Refrigerator Chart

People following the MIND diet have expressed great satisfaction with the simplicity of our tracking system, as illustrated by the MIND Diet Refrigerator Chart shown on page 136. As you might have guessed from the name "Refrigerator Chart," the intention is to keep this tracking tool visible right where eating and meal preparation would take place—the kitchen! We encourage you to make copies of the chart or download a copy from TheOfficialMINDdiet.com and post it on your refrigerator to keep track of your intake throughout the week. Start with a fresh chart each week, then simply keep a tally of the servings of foods for each day. It's a really easy way to see how your eating patterns stack up against your risk for Alzheimer's disease. Week 1 of the program will invite you to begin using the Refrigerator Chart to see what your current intake of the MIND foods is like. If you'd like to get a head start on this, you can try the following exercise.

We cannot overemphasize the power of this simple tool when it comes to setting yourself up for success in the program. Its first aim is to bring awareness to your eating habits even before you decide to change anything. It may sound a bit strange to begin a healthy eating program by *not* making initial changes, but as mentioned previously, our goal in this program is to teach you *how to eat*, rather than just to tell you *what to eat*. This begins with taking inventory. You probably wouldn't try to make changes to a project without assessing the

---

MIND DIET REFRIGERATOR CHART

INSTRUCTIONS: For the first week, don't change any of your eating habits. Follow the steps below to track all MIND diet *Foods to Choose* and *Foods to Limit* using the MIND Diet Refrigerator Chart.

1. Tally or write in the number of MIND food servings you eat for each food daily. Write a "0" if you did not eat that food on a specific day.
2. At the end of the week, add up and fill in the Total MIND Servings in the column provided, then check the MIND Food Points column and fill in the MIND Points column for each food (1, 0.5, or 0).
3. At the end of the week, add up the total number of MIND Points for all foods and enter it in the MIND Diet Score box at the bottom of the chart.
4. Check the RESEARCH SHOWS box to see if your MIND Diet Score falls in the range associated with a reduction in risk for Alzheimer's disease.
5. Start over with a blank chart the following week and write your previous week's MIND Diet Score at the top of the new chart to monitor your progress.

---

current status of the project. Likewise, gaining full awareness of your eating habits before trying to change anything will help you determine what needs to change—and what doesn't. Many people begin lifestyle programs by trying to change several things at once without the recommendation to notice the impact of the modifications. For example, a common misconception is that sweets are not allowed on a "diet," and it can be easy to get into the mindset of trying to banish all sweets from your routine. With self-monitoring, you may be surprised to learn that you are not eating an excess of sweets to begin with. You may even notice that things could be added instead of subtracted to make your eating habits healthier, such as leafy green vegetables or berries.

Week of: _____

FOODS TO CHOOSE	M	T	W	Th	F	Sa	Su	Total MIND Servings This Week
Leafy Green Vegetables (LG) **Goal:** 1 serving/day **Serving size:** 1 cup raw or ½ cup cooked								
Other Vegetables (OV) **Goal:** 1 serving/day **Serving size:** ½ cup, cooked or raw								
Berries (Ber) **Goal:** 5 servings/week **Serving size:** ½ cup								
Extra-Virgin Olive Oil (EVOO) **Goal:** 2 servings/day **Serving size:** 1 tablespoon								
Nuts & Seeds (Nut) **Goal:** 5 servings/week **Serving size:** 1 ounce nuts or seeds or 2 tablespoons nut/seed butter								
Fish & Seafood (Fsh) **Goal:** 1 serving/week **Serving size:** 3–5 ounces								
Poultry (Poul) **Goal:** 2 servings/week **Serving size:** 3–5 ounces without skin/bones								
Whole Grains (WG) **Goal:** 3 servings/day **Serving size:** 1 slice bread or ½ cup cooked grains								
Beans & Legumes (Bn) **Goal:** 3 servings/week **Serving size:** ½ cup canned or cooked								
Wine (Win) **Goal:** 1 serving/day **Serving size:** 5 fluid ounces								

Last Week's MIND Score: _____

MIND Food Points		MIND Points (1, 0.5, or 0)
0–2 servings/week	0	
3–6 servings/week	0.5	
7+ servings/week	1	
0–4 servings/week	0	
5–6 servings/week	0.5	
7+ servings/week	1	
0 servings/week	0	
1–4 servings/week	0.5	
5+ servings/week	1	
0–6 servings/week	0	
7–13 servings/week	0.5	
14+ servings/week	1	
0 servings/week	0	
1–4 servings/week	0.5	
5+ servings/week	1	
0 servings/week	0	
1+ servings/week	1	
0 servings/week	0	
1 serving/week	0.5	
2+ servings/week	1	
0–4 servings/week	0	
5–20 servings/week	0.5	
21+ servings/week	1	
0 servings/week	0	
1–2 servings/week	0.5	
3+ servings/week	1	
0 servings/week	0	
1–6 servings/week	0.5	
7 servings/week	1	
8+ servings/week	0	

FOODS TO LIMIT	M	T	W	Th	F	Sa	Su	Total MIND Servings This Week
Red Meat & Processed Meat (RM) **Goal:** 0–3 servings/week **Serving size:** 3–5 ounces								
Butter & Stick Margarine (But) **Goal:** 0–1 serving/day **Serving size:** 1 teaspoon								
Full-Fat Cheese (Chs) **Goal:** 0–2 servings/week **Serving size:** 1 ounce								
Fried Foods (Fri) **Goal:** 0–1 serving/week **Serving size:** 1 serving								
Sweets, Pastries & Sweet Drinks (Swt) **Goal:** 0–4 servings/week **Serving size:** 1 treat or 8-ounce drink								

RESEARCH SHOWS:	0–6.5	7.0–8.0	8.5–12.5	13–15
People who had a MIND Diet Score of . . . had a reduced risk for developing Alzheimer's disease by . . .	No Reduced Risk	35% Reduced Risk	53% Reduced Risk	Potentially Greatest Reduced Risk*

*Assumed based on linear association between MIND scores and cognitive outcomes.

MIND Food Points		MIND Points (1, 0.5, or 0)
0–3 servings/week	1	
4–6 servings/week	0.5	
7+ servings/week	0	
0–7 servings/week	1	
8–13 servings/week	0.5	
14+ servings/week	0	
0–2 servings/week	1	
3–6 servings/week	0.5	
7+ servings/week	0	
0–1 serving/week	1	
2–3 servings/week	0.5	
4+ servings/week	0	
0–4 servings/week	1	
5–6 servings/week	0.5	
7+ servings/week	0	

This Week's MIND Diet Score: _____

All information is useful, and self-monitoring will help you take an objective look at the facts before trying to make changes. Be your own detective to determine how your habits measure up against the MIND guidelines.

MEAL PLANNING

The next SMART MIND habit for success in this program is all about meal planning. We consider this to be the "lean meat and sweet potatoes" of the whole program. It has to do with scheduling and planning. Another way to look at it is managing your time. In our modern day of cell phones and instant entertainment at our fingertips, we are overwhelmed to the point where we don't have time to do basic things—like self-care through meal planning and preparation. This is an important topic. Stephen Covey, author of the best-selling book *The 7 Habits of Highly Effective People*, suggests that the first habit required for making big changes is to prioritize, which boils down to time management.

The truth is that there are only 24 hours in a day, and balancing the demands of family, work, spiritual life, friends, social events, community service, self-care, and health can be stressful. This is a time to evaluate where your time is being spent, because in the end, you make time for what's important. That may look like missing social gatherings or work events so you can take time to exercise and grocery shop for healthy foods. Or it may mean skipping the morning Facebook or Instagram scroll so you can do 20 minutes of journaling or meditation. Over time, you will find that the more you nurture yourself through healthy practices, the more you will be able to give to your loved ones and to your passions because you will have the energy and clarity to be present.

Tool #2: Calendar with Reminders

The next tool you will need is a calendar to schedule three key weekly activities: menu planning, grocery shopping, and meal preparation. The calendar ideally should allow you to see both a weekly and monthly view. Perhaps you already use an e-calendar or have an app on your smartphone. Or maybe you're a busy parent making efforts to keep the household organized with a shared calendar of chores, events, sports, and school activities. Whether an electronic calendar or a physical paper book, whiteboard, or journal, it really is about what works for you. This can be your opportunity to customize a tool in your toolbox to make it fun.

One key component is to ensure a method for reminders within your scheduling system. This can be one reason online or smartphone app calendars are useful since you can program reminders in advance. Otherwise, we recommend some sort of visual system for reminders such as sticky notes or even a separate phone or watch alarm with programmed reminders to alert you to important tasks. We recommend having reminders when you first get started creating new habits, so it is more than just wishful thinking.

"A goal without a plan is just a wish."

—Unknown

Week 1 of the program will prompt you to begin using your Calendar with Reminders to schedule your new habits. Whatever system you choose, be sure to merge your *other* scheduled priorities with these healthy lifestyle priorities. The goal is to blend healthy eating into your existing lifestyle routine. The calendar on the next page gives an example.

The calendar shown represents activities for an entire month, and it's meant to be fluid—just as the events in our lives are constantly changing. The bolded events are the new habits of menu planning, grocery shopping, and meal preparation merged with the non-bolded existing events such as kids' sports practices and games, exercise

August

Sun	Mon	Tue	Wed	Thu	Fri	Sat
30 8a Grocery Shop & Meal Prep/ Clean Fridge	**31**	**1** 5p Soccer Practice	**2** 7p Meditation	**3**	**4** 6p Dinner Out	**5** 8:30a Spin Class 10a Menu Plan 12p Soccer Game
6 8a Grocery Shop & Meal Prep/ Clean Fridge	**7**	**8** 5p Soccer Practice	**9** 7p Meditation	**10**	**11** 6:30p Sitter 7p Dinner Out w/Neighbors	**12** 8:30a Spin Class 10a Menu Plan
13 8a Grocery Shop & Meal Prep/ Clean Fridge	**14**	**15** 5p Grocery Shop for Party ~~5p Soccer Practice~~	**16** 5p Meal Prep for Party ~~7p Meditation~~	**17** 7p Baking	**18** ~~5p Dinner Out~~ 7p Party Prep	**19** ~~8:30a Spin Class~~ ~~10a Menu Plan~~ 12p Birthday Party
20 7a Pick Recipes, Grocery Shop, & Meal Prep/ Clean Fridge	**21**	**22** 5p Soccer Practice	**23** 7p Meditation	**24** 5p Board Meeting 6p Leftovers	**25** 6p Dinner Out	**26** 8:30a Spin Class 10a Menu Plan 12p Soccer Game
27 8a Grocery Shop ~~& Meal Prep /Clean Fridge~~ 11a Charity Event	**28** 5p Meal Prep/Clean Fridge	**29** 5p Soccer Practice	**30** 7p Meditation	**31**		

classes, parties, nights out, and volunteer events. It can be helpful to map out these repeated new habits for several weeks in advance so you can see them at a glance in the monthly calendar view.

If you're someone who already feels overscheduled, be realistic with yourself and acknowledge that some things in your current routine will have to shift if you expect the new habits to "stick." That doesn't have to mean giving up eating out or abandoning your extracurricular activities. However, it may mean prioritizing some new activities if you expect them to develop into habits and being flexible with some existing activities when special events pop up. Prioritizing means choosing which event is more important to fill that slot, but also choosing to move a competing priority to another day and time, rather than delete it entirely. This is just one example of how planning ahead and allowing for flexibility with scheduling can set you up for success with meal planning.

For new habits, it's best to choose the same day and time each week to increase the likelihood of bringing the habit to automaticity.

You may want to set an alert in your phone or put the calendar some-where visible so that you will not forget to do these activities. When you get into a routine of doing something on the same day and at the same time each week, the reward will be feelings of preparedness and accomplishment, fueling the motivation to continue the new habit. Eventually, you will begin to engage in these habits without the need to schedule them in your calendar.

If you're not used to scheduling in a system like this, then even the act of maintaining your weekly calendar becomes a new habit. This means you will need to practice. Our advice for you here is to be patient with yourself. Organization looks different for everyone. Just do your best to take it one day at a time.

Tool #3: Menu Plan and Recipe Bank

Setting Up Your Menu Plan Schedule

After carving out the time on your calendar to plan your menu, you can plug in some actual meal ideas to get into the habit of meal plan-ning. This idea of scheduling meals into a calendar *is* meal planning, so if you've never done it before, it may be easier than you think! It is best to begin by looking ahead to any events, meetings, activities, or dinner invites you may already have scheduled in the upcoming week. If you are going of town or have a night planned out with friends, for instance, you will need to plan around those days/meals. If you have a late meeting or kid's school event, you may want to opt for an easy meal or leftovers that night.

To simplify planning for specific menu items, you might begin with just one meal. If you're a breakfast skipper who would like to try a new habit of eating breakfast regularly, you could schedule breakfast on your calendar daily or most days. You may also need a reminder on the calendar to alert you to eat at breakfast time. For many Americans, dinner is the most significant meal and therefore requires the most thought. If you have a large family to feed, you can double or triple the amount you make and plan for the same meal to appear as leftovers on the calendar—even if the meal is slightly different the following night. We also recommend having a go-to recipe that can be thrown together with minimal effort on the days when you're short on time, preferably something that uses pantry items you keep in stock. Chickpea Tuna Salad (page 273) and Olive Oil Veggie Scramble (page 243), for instance, are both delicious, quick meals that are packed with nutrients. You should also spend some time infusing a little fun into the calendar. Theme nights—like Soup Sunday, Meatless Monday, or Taco Tuesday—are great ways to keep things interesting, prevent boredom, and get the family involved in choosing some mealtime options.

Cooking at home every night is not realistic for most people, so aim for 3 or 4 nights per week to make home-prepared dinners. A sample week could look like this: 3 or 4 nights preparing dinner at home, 2 nights of leftovers, 1 or 2 nights eating out or taking in. Find a rhythm that works for you and your household. You can post your menu plan on your refrigerator or kitchen bulletin board so everyone in the household can see the plans for the week, including what's for dinner. If you have picky eaters, enlist their help with at least one meal each week. If they choose the meal, they may be more likely to feel empowered and less likely to be picky about eating it. You can build a database of your weekly menus by simply taking a picture of your calendar or saving a printed copy in a folder or electronically on your computer. This way, you can keep track of the menu items you liked and disliked for the following weeks. You'll start setting up a menu plan as early as week 1 in the 6-week program.

What If I Don't Cook?

A common perceived barrier to developing healthier eating habits is feeling like you "don't cook." To maximize possibilities and minimize stress with meal planning, we recommend throwing the word *cook* out of your vocabulary—at least at first. It's much less intimidating to think about "preparing" or "assembling" meals at home versus "cooking." Don't worry if you have limited experience in the kitchen—at the very least, you have the ideas presented in this book. That is more than enough to start your Recipe Bank. Perhaps even the word *recipe* is intimidating to you. If that's the case, think of recipes more as meal ideas. You don't need to identify every meal you will eat ahead of time. Aiming for two or three recipe or meal ideas is plenty to begin. And you can always flip back to part II for a plethora of "In a Routine" or "In a Rush" suggestions that do not require written recipes or a lot of time or effort.

Building Your Recipe Bank

One way to stay motivated with healthy eating is to incorporate new recipes to build your Recipe Bank. While it's great to have go-to favorite meals, we can sometimes get stuck in a rut. Consider the following strategies for experimenting with new recipes:

- Check out cookbooks from the library on cuisines you enjoy or would like to learn more about, such as Italian, Indian, Peruvian, or Thai.

- Follow food bloggers on social media platforms such as Instagram, Pinterest, or Facebook.

- Host a potluck get-together and invite guests to bring components of a meal (mains, salads, sides, and desserts *or* vegetables, carbs, proteins).

We will invite you to begin incorporating recipes into the menu planning process in week 3 of the 6-week program.

For a deep dive into the meal-planning process and to access an interactive, downloadable meal planner bonus tool with sample menu ideas, visit TheOfficialMINDdiet.com.

Tool #4: Grocery Shopping and Meal Preparation Plan

When it comes to meal planning, having a plan for grocery shopping and meal preparation is a must! After completing the simple act of scheduling these activities into your calendar among your existing events, you'll be one step ahead.

Grocery Shopping

Before you head out to the grocery store, there are a few things you can do to set yourself up for success. Here are some best practices for navigating the grocery store:

Start by "shopping" your own kitchen. First, determine what foods you have that need to be used up or that you could use as ingredients for meals for the upcoming week. Using what you have is one of the most cost-effective, eco-friendly methods for meal planning. If you have beans, rice, and vegetables, for instance, you could mix up a "Sunday stew" to provide two or even three meals or side dishes for the week. Also, take this time to clean your refrigerator of any expired food. Having a clean, organized refrigerator makes everything easier and more appealing to eat.

Always shop with a grocery list. The list will be generated from ingredients for meals on your calendar and any recipe ideas you've chosen. Organize your list according to the grocery store layout—produce (leafy greens, other vegetables, berries, other fruits), proteins (fish, poultry), pantry items (EVOO, whole grains, beans, nuts), and refrigerated and frozen items (milk, low-fat cheese, eggs, frozen veggies, frozen berries).

For a downloadable grocery list template, visit TheOfficialMIND diet.com.

Never go to the grocery store hungry. This will prevent you from buying things that aren't on your list, which will be beneficial for your waistline and your wallet. It can also be helpful to try to go at times when the store is less crowded, perhaps earlier in the morning or later in the evenings. Your shopping may be more enjoyable, and you may be able to be more MINDful in your food purchases. Another option is to consider grocery delivery services such as Instacart or Amazon Fresh. This can help eliminate impulse purchases and cut down on shopping time if your schedule is tight.

Don't be fooled by advertising—read your food labels. Most of the foods we recommend are fresh and thus do not require a label, which is a good indication of nutritious food in its most natural form. When you are purchasing food with a label, look at the ingredients list, as this is the best indicator of what you are consuming. After you look at the ingredients list, look at the Nutrition Facts label to better understand what nutrients you are eating. There is a lot of information on nutrition labels, which makes it more difficult to understand how to eat healthy and make simple food choices for you and your family. Following is a quick breakdown for you as a consumer to understand key label components.

Nutrition Facts

8 servings per container

Serving size   2/3 cup (55g)

Amount per serving

Calories   230

	% Daily Value*
Total Fat 8g	**10%**
Saturated Fat 1g	**5%**
Trans Fat 0g	
Cholesterol 0mg	**0%**
Sodium 160mg	**7%**
Total Carbohydrate 37g	**13%**
Dietary Fiber 4g	**14%**
Total Sugars 12g	
Includes 10g Added Sugars	**20%**
Protein 3g	
Vitamin D 2mcg	10%
Calcium 260mg	20%
Iron 8mg	45%
Potassium 240mg	6%

* The % Daily Value (DV) tells you how much a nutrient in a serving of food contributes to a daily diet. 2,000 calories a day is used for general nutrition advice.

For the purposes of this discussion, we ask you to ignore the % Daily Value (%DV) along the right side of the label, as well as the vitamin and mineral information at the bottom. This is just to allow you to focus on the most pertinent information. You really need to focus on only a small amount of information to empower you to make informed, healthy choices.

Remember that these are general guidelines and should not be interpreted as a prescribed diet. Always check with your doctor before following a prescribed diet or see a registered dietitian for guidance.

Serving size: Because there can be multiple servings per container, it's important to know how much you're eating compared to how much is in the entire package.

Calories: Depending upon your individual caloric needs and activity level, a target daily goal may be 300 to 600 calories per meal and 150 to 300 calories per snack.
Quick Tip: If you're not into calorie counting (which we generally don't recommend for most people—at least not long-term), you may want to take a more intuitive approach to healthy eating and energy balance by aiming to prepare meals at home most days and to make half of your lunch and dinner meals leafy green and/or other vegetables.

Total Fat: The quality or type of fat is of interest when interpreting the Total Fat on a Nutrition Facts label. Total Fat includes both healthy fats (mono- and polyunsaturated fats) and unhealthy fats (saturated fat and trans fat).
Quick Tip: Aim for no more than 3 grams saturated fat and 0 grams trans fat per serving.

Cholesterol: We don't encourage you to pay much attention to this. Instead, focus on saturated fat, since it plays a much larger role in increasing your blood cholesterol (and overall health risk) than dietary cholesterol.

Sodium: About one-third of Americans are sensitive to too much sodium in the diet, which means that those who consume sodium in excess may experience high blood pressure. In general, salt = sodium.
Always check with your doctor for personalized recommendations based on your own health risk profile, but daily sodium recommendations are typically 1,500 milligrams or less if you have high

blood pressure or take blood pressure medication and no more than 2,300 milligrams if you have normal blood pressure.

Quick Tip: A general rule of thumb can be to look for meals with no more than 600 milligrams sodium and snacks with no more than 300 milligrams. By law, a low-sodium food has no more than 140 milligrams sodium per serving.

Total Carbohydrate: Keeping Total Carbohydrate at a moderate level can help you maintain a healthy weight, which may reduce your risk for heart disease, type 2 diabetes, and memory loss. We also know that the type of carbohydrate is key, with refined white grains and added sugars being most harmful for the brain.

Quick Tip: A good starting point for Total Carbohydrate is 30 to 60 grams for meals and 15 to 30 grams for snacks. A good food source of fiber contains 3 grams of Dietary Fiber.

Protein: Protein is essential to building and maintaining muscle mass. It is ideal to consume a combination of healthy carbohydrates with protein, since carbohydrates give us energy, and protein sustains that energy. Protein also helps keep us feeling full. Many people feel hungry after meals if they do not consume adequate protein or find themselves with cravings later in the day.

Quick Tip: Aim for meals with at least 20 grams of protein and snacks with at least 5 grams.

Plan to Meal Prep

Prioritizing your meal prep plan and incorporating it into your weekly routine is key. Again, the first step is to actually carve out the time to do this. Many people find it easiest to do meal prep the same day as grocery shopping so they can get started on it while putting away groceries.

The goal is to prep as much as you can up to 3 or 4 days ahead to help streamline your routine throughout the week. This could include chopping vegetables, preparing sauces and salad dressings, marinating meat, hard-boiling eggs, and cooking grains that can all be stored in the refrigerator. Put prepared food for the same dishes in containers stacked together so they are easier to grab.

You will likely need to refresh your veggies and would not want to prep all your meals too far ahead or they won't taste fresh, so you may want to schedule in an additional day of meal prep. Alternatively, you may find that prep happens naturally as you are making other meals in real time. In week 4 of the 6-week program, we encourage you to generate a plan for meal prep ahead of time to make day-of cooking more efficient. As this habit strengthens, you'll fall into a natural rhythm to stay one step ahead.

Tool #5: MIND Plate for Meal Planning

Even when you have a good understanding of the MIND diet *Foods to Choose* and *Foods to Limit*, it still requires a bit of thinking ahead to plan healthy meals. At first it can seem overwhelming to have to plan your entire week in advance, so we are introducing a strategy here to bring balance to your meals one "plate" at a time.

The MIND Plate for Meal Planning provides a visual guide for how to build meals with brain-healthy foods according to the categories we discussed in part II—vegetables and fruit, proteins, carbohydrates, and fats. By week 5 of the program, you'll be using the MIND Plate to build balanced meals with the MIND foods. If you'd like to get a head start on this, you can try the following exercise.

MIND PLATE FOR MEAL PLANNING

INSTRUCTIONS:

1. Fill ½ plate (about the size of 2 fists) with leafy greens and other nonstarchy vegetables; you can include berries too, if you like.
2. Fill ¼ plate (about the size of 1 palm) with lean protein, such as poultry or fish.
3. Fill ¼ plate (about the size of 1 fist) with healthy carbs, such as whole grains and/or beans.
4. Add fats (about the size of 1 or 2 thumbs) in the form of unsaturated fats such as EVOO or nuts/seeds.

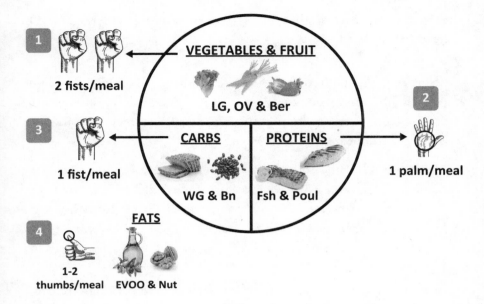

I invite you to reframe the way you think about meals. Rather than just planning to eat "breakfast" or "dinner" foods, challenge yourself to think about the quality of the entire meal, including the portions within each food category and how they come together to form an overall balanced meal. As a reminder, the food categories are as follows:

1. **Vegetables & Fruit** (LG, OV, Ber [leafy green vegetables, other vegetables, berries])

2. **Proteins** (Poul, Fsh [poultry, fish & seafood])

3. **Carbs** (WG, Bn [whole grains, beans & legumes])

4. **Fats** (EVOO, Nut [extra-virgin olive oil, nuts & seeds])

Portion control is an important part of meal planning. Let's begin by distinguishing a *serving* from a *portion*, as we will continue to use these terms distinctly in the context of meal planning with the MIND Plate going forward.

> **Serving:** A standardized amount of food. Examples: 1 slice whole-grain bread, 2 tablespoons nut butter, ½ cup berries, 1 cup leafy greens, ½ cup cut-up other vegetables such as carrots, 1 tablespoon EVOO
>
> **Portion:** The amount of food one chooses to eat in a meal or snack. Examples: 2 slices whole-grain bread, 2 tablespoons nut butter, 1 cup raspberries (½ cup smashed, ½ cup whole), 2 cups spinach or mixed greens, ¼ cup shredded carrots, 1 tablespoon EVOO

In the above example, a variety of MIND food servings are presented from a lunch of a peanut butter and smashed berry sandwich with a leafy green salad on the side. For some food categories, it's perfectly acceptable to have more than 1 *serving* in the overall *portion* of that category. For example, 1 serving of whole grains is equivalent to 1 slice of bread, but for a sandwich, the natural portion would be 2 slices, which equates to 2 servings. Since the goal for whole grains is 3 servings each day, it may be desirable to get in more than 1 serving in a single meal.

In contrast, you may not get in a full serving in one portion of the meal. For example, a typical side salad may have a sprinkling of shredded carrots on top, which isn't quite a full serving. Whenever you think that there isn't quite enough of something to make a full serving, simply track it as a ½ serving for that meal.

A great tool for estimating portion sizes for the MIND Plate is to use your hands, literally! (See the illustration above.) Let's break it down to best understand how it works.

Step 1 is to begin at the top of the plate to plan for vegetables and fruit (but mostly vegetables).

> **ReMINDer:** Berries are the only fruit included on the MIND diet. Fill the MIND diet plate with mostly vegetables.

The goal for berries is a total of five ½-cup servings per week compared to a combined total of 14 servings of leafy greens and other vegetables weekly. This food category should make up about 50 percent of the meal, or about the size of 2 "fists." The average person's 2 fists is equivalent to about 2 cups leafy greens/veggies or a combo of 1 cup leafy greens/veggies plus about 1 cup berries. A common household comparator for 2 fists would be 2 baseballs.

Step 2 is to add a lean protein to the meal. Lean proteins include poultry, such as skinless chicken or turkey breast, and any fish that is not deep-fried. Remember that the goal for poultry is twice weekly, whereas the goal for fish and seafood is just once weekly. This food category should make up about 25 percent of the plate, or about the size of 1 "palm." The average person's palm (without fingers) is about the same size as 3 to 5 ounces of cooked protein, but this could vary greatly, so this is a food category for which I highly recommend paying attention to the serving size. You may need more protein and overall calories for your weight, height, and physical activity levels. A common household item for size comparison for 3 ounces of cooked poultry or fish and seafood is a standard deck of playing cards. If you're someone who has a bigger build or is very active, a portion larger than a deck of cards may be appropriate in one sitting.

> **ReMINDers:** Chicken and turkey are best consumed as skinless white (breast) meat, not fried.
>
> The richest sources of fish containing omega-3s are salmon, albacore tuna, sardines, anchovies, and mackerel.

Step 3 in the process of building balanced meals with the MIND Plate is to add some healthy carbs in the form of whole grains or beans/legumes. Since the frequency goal is much higher for whole grains (3 times per day) than for beans (3 times per week), it is likely that this section will be filled more often with whole grains than with beans. In either case, it is recommended that this food fill about 25 percent of the plate or 1 "fist" in physical size. A common household item for comparison in this food category would be 1 baseball.

> **ReMINDer:** Whole grains such as pasta and rice double or even triple in size after cooking. Be sure to portion whole grains onto the MIND Plate *after* cooking.

After balancing vegetables and fruit, proteins, and carbs on the MIND Plate, **step 4** in the meal planning process is to add fats. The key here is to aim for unsaturated fats. And luckily, this is also the secret to creating a meal with delicious flavor. Fat is one of the things that contributes to enhancing the flavor of foods, so choosing healthy fats is the perfect recipe for keeping our brains and our bellies healthy and happy. In addition to the MIND diet foods of extra-virgin olive oil and nuts and seeds, other sources of healthy unsaturated fats include fatty fish, avocados, and whole olives.

Some ideas for incorporating these healthy fats include using EVOO as a base to make delicious sauces and dressings to drizzle on top of vegetables and grains. EVOO is versatile and can be combined with different vinegars, citruses, spices, and herbs to create balanced, vibrant sauces. You may also choose to lightly sauté your vegetables with EVOO to boost polyphenol content and enhance flavor.

Fats are also important to help absorption of fat-soluble vitamins and antioxidants in the vegetables and grains you are consuming. Nuts and seeds are included in the brain-healthy fats category; they can be toasted, chopped, and blended into sauces. Keep in mind that the goal for frequency of EVOO (2 tablespoons daily) is much higher than for nuts (5 ounces weekly), so you'll likely be choosing EVOO more often.

Because the foods in this category are very calorie-dense, the recommendation for a total portion is 1 to 2 "thumbs" per meal. This equates to 1 to 2 servings of EVOO (1 serving = 1 tablespoon) and ½ to 1 serving of nuts and seeds (1 serving = 1 ounce nuts/seeds or 2 tablespoons nut/seed butter). A simpler way to estimate the portion for this food category would be to compare it to a golf ball.

ReMINDer: Unsaturated fats are one of the most potent food categories to benefit the brain. They are also very calorie dense.

2 tablespoons EVOO = 240 calories

1 ounce nuts/seeds or 2 tablespoons nut/seed butter = ~200 calories

If you are trying to lose weight, be sure to carefully measure EVOO and nut portions when planning for balanced MIND meals.

So, where do the *Foods to Limit* fit on the MIND Plate for Meal Planning? Each of these five foods will fit *within* another food category on the MIND Plate. They all have saturated fat in common so will primarily go in the fats category, but many of them will also be included in another category as well. Let's take a look at the *Foods to Limit*:

1. **Red Meat and Processed Meat:** 3–5 ounces, 0–3 times/week **(FATS + PROTEINS)**

2. **Butter and Stick Margarine:** 1 teaspoon, 0–7 times/week **(FATS)**

3. **Full-Fat Cheese:** 1 ounce, 0–2 times/week **(FATS)**

4. **Fried Foods:** 1 meal, 0–1 time/week **(FATS + PROTEINS or CARBS)**

5. **Sweets, Pastries, and Sweet Drinks:** 1 treat or 8-ounce drink, 0–4 times/week **(FATS + CARBS)**

Butter and stick margarine and full-fat cheese are made up of mostly fat, so they will fit just within the fats on the MIND Plate. That means you would want to balance these foods with any other fats planned for the same meal when incorporating one or more of the *Foods to Limit* to keep the overall meal balanced. For example, if you've planned a meal of a leafy green salad that includes an EVOO-based dressing, along with whole-grain pasta with peanut sauce, you may want to choose a different appetizer than cheese and crackers, since you've already "fulfilled" the fat category. In this example, something like a shrimp cocktail could fit nicely, since the addition of a protein would round out the MIND Plate.

For the times you will be enjoying the *Foods to Limit*, some of them will spill over into other areas on the plate. For example, if you plan to eat red meat or fried foods, such as a burger or fried chicken, you will want to consider this in both the fats and the proteins categories. If you have french fries with the burger or chicken or choose to have dessert, you may also want to reduce the overall portion of the carbs section of your plate in order to maintain a healthy balance, especially if you're trying to lose weight. As always, whenever consuming any of the moderation foods, you may want to simply remember to exercise portion control and make good use of the refrigerator chart tracking tool to ensure you're staying within the weekly limits for the saturated fat group as a whole.

For the purposes of bringing clarity on how to use the MIND Plate for Meal Planning tool, we've been pretty detailed in our explanation above! But please remember that you are not actually "dieting." We recommend focusing on the weekly target for each individual food and staying MINDful of your intake throughout the week to follow the MIND guidelines with ease. Not everything has to be perfect.

One of the most beloved features of the diet is that no individual food or food category is completely off limits. Although it may be tough to keep all five foods within the recommended targets, you can still get a therapeutic MIND diet score even if there is a category

> **ReMINDer:** All the items on the MIND diet *Foods to Limit* list are high in saturated fat, believed to cause oxidative damage and inflammation in the brain.
>
> Be MINDful of portions for these items and consume in moderation by balancing with other MIND foods using the MIND Diet Refrigerator Chart.

target you are unable to meet or *choose* not to meet. Remember that even people who followed the diet only moderately well saw some benefit in terms of slowed cognitive decline and reduced risk for Alzheimer's disease. Who says you can't have your cake and eat it too? To reinforce the new habit of creating balanced meals, you can practice using the MIND Plate for Meal Planning one meal at a time or integrate it earlier in your meal planning to ensure you are choosing balanced recipes for the week.

Bonus Tips: Healthy Eating While Traveling and at Restaurants

Although traveling and eating in restaurants isn't a component of meal planning per se, it does require a bit of planning ahead to make healthy choices while on the go. Eating while traveling often presents challenges, as you are at the mercy of restaurants, hotels, and roadside or airport food—yikes! We all want to be able to enjoy delicious cuisine while traveling and still feed ourselves with foods that protect our brain and heart. Here are some helpful tips and tricks to love your body and brain while on the road:

1. *Try to eat as you normally would for at least 1 or 2 meals of the day.* If you typically eat oatmeal and blueberries for breakfast, then eggs with bacon may not be the best choice for your body. Pick a few meals each day that closely resemble what you eat at home.

2. *Choose snacks that combine carbs and protein.* Airports have come a long way in their snack food department. If you are looking to grab a snack or something to help you get through a flight, choose items that combine healthy carbs and protein. Think hummus and pretzels with a hard-boiled egg, an apple with a small pack of nuts, or crackers with peanut butter. If you're on a road trip, try to pack healthy snacks and sandwiches such as peanut butter and honey on whole-grain bread or turkey wraps with veggies and fruit.

3. *Pay attention to cooking techniques.* Fried, battered, and sautéed methods use a good dose of fat from either butter or oil (most likely not EVOO) and are in the category of *Foods to Limit*. Broiled, baked, roasted, grilled, poached, or steamed dishes are usually lighter.

4. *Be aware of creamy dressings and sauces.* Sauces add calories, often from fat. Ask for dressings and sauces on the side so you can control how much you eat.

5. *Order a side salad with your meal or swap french fries for a side of veggies.* This can help you get in your leafy greens and other vegetables and prevent overeating the *Foods to Limit*.

6. *Look for Mediterranean (such as Lebanese, Israeli, Greek, or Turkish) restaurants when you are traveling on the road or in a new city.* These cuisines often have vegetable-centered dishes that will align with your MIND diet goals.

7. *Plan for non-restaurant meals.* See if the local coffee shop has healthy options such as nuts or a fruit cup with Greek yogurt. Or pick up a premade salad from the local grocery store. You can also pack instant oatmeal for a quick, light breakfast to get in some whole grains.

8. *Enjoy your meals without overindulging.* Ask for half portions, order à la carte, or ask for a take-home container with your

meal and put half away before you begin eating to prevent overeating.

9. *Be MINDful of alcohol and sugar-sweetened beverages.* Drink water as much as possible, and when you do drink alcohol, aim to limit your intake to 1 drink per day.

ACTION PLANNING

We've all heard that setting goals, and then working to achieve them, is the most effective path to success. Our next SMART MIND habit for success will help you break down your goals into practical steps.

Tool #6: Small Goals List

An action plan is composed of a set of *small* goals, distinct from long-term goals. The best way to achieve a long-term goal is to break it down into small goals pursued consistently over time.

First, get clear on your long-term goal. If you've chosen this book, perhaps your goal is to reduce your risk for dementia or to lose weight—or both. In that case, you may decide on a long-term goal to sustain an average MIND diet score between 13 and 15 most weeks and perhaps have an ideal weight goal in mind for yourself. Once you have a good understanding of your long-term goal, then you can break it down into smaller, action-oriented steps—what we think of as "small goals"—that will be the means to the end.

Next, choose just a few small goals in your overall action plan. The process of self-monitoring with your refrigerator chart and the other meal-planning activities, such as scheduling with your calendar and selecting your recipes, will reveal areas of focus for these goals, such as whether you need to improve on targets for specific MIND foods, prioritize healthy habits around social events, or figure out what types of meals you may want to plan for the upcoming week.

It's best to begin with just two or three goals, especially if you are just getting started with a lifestyle change.

It's important to ensure that your small goals are SMART. Yep, we love this acronym! In this context, "SMART" is a well-known framework used for both professional and personal goal achievement. Each goal you set should fulfill these five requirements:

Specific: The goal outlines a particular component of what you'd like to improve. So, if you want to improve your habit of vegetable intake, a specific goal might target a way to increase consumption of leafy green vegetables.

Measurable: The goal can be described in a quantifiable way, so that progress can be tracked. A measurable goal might be to eat leafy greens every day, since the MIND diet's weekly target for leafy greens is 7 servings per week.

Action-Based: The goal has some action or behavior tied to it. In other words, this part of the goal includes "the how." An action-based goal for increasing leafy greens might be to serve a salad with dinner every night.

Realistic: Think about how likely it is that you will achieve your goal on a scale of 1 to 10. Rating your confidence will help you determine if the goal is appropriate. If you answered 6 or lower, you may want to modify this goal to something that you can be more confident about achieving. For example, it may be tough to incorporate a salad with dinner *every* night, so you could aim for 4 nights a week instead of 7.

Time-Based: The goal has a timeframe attached to it. The framework we've set up for you in the 6-week program should make this one pretty easy, since we will be encouraging you to think of your habits in weekly increments. A time-based goal might be to aim for a leafy green salad with dinner 4 out of 7 nights over the next week.

The final step is to make a list of the small goals to form the overall action plan—and post the plan somewhere visible. This could be on your calendar, since you'll likely be looking at that daily, on a bulletin board, or even just on a sticky note on your computer monitor. Some people get creative and take a photo of the goals to use as the background picture for their phone to remind them each time they look at their phone. Just like most things in this program, this is an opportunity for you to customize what works best for you.

Think about what long-term and small goals might look like for you. This will be good practice before beginning the 6-week program, when we will be offering suggestions for small goals and then asking you to set a weekly action plan. It'll also give you a chance to experiment with what lifestyle habits may—or may not—be sustainable. If you'd like to practice with the habit of action planning before beginning the program, you can try the following exercise.

ACTION PLANNING

INSTRUCTIONS:

1. Define a long-term goal.
2. Choose two or three small goals.
3. Confirm that each of your small goals is SMART (see page 160).
4. Write out your Small Goals List to form your action plan and post it somewhere visible.

REFLECTION

The next SMART MIND habit for success is reflection. Reflection consists of taking the time to think about your intentions and actions, and the results you get back. This can be done by considering the successes and challenges you have with your small goals throughout the week and actively evaluating how you make decisions when things are going well or when challenges arise. This allows you to gain the insight necessary to reinforce good habits and correct poor ones.

For example, you may notice that when you go to bed by 10 p.m., you avoid snacking at night, wake well rested, have an energizing breakfast, and make time to be physically active—all resulting in a much more productive day. The insight: going to bed earlier is more aligned with your overall intentions for health and well-being.

You may also find that when you have a stressful day at work, you skip your workout and go home to drink wine and order takeout. This reflection may help you realize that when you are stressed, you seek out the comfort of alcohol and junk food. In that case, you might modify or add a small goal to plan ahead for healthier ways to calm your body and mind, such as going for a walk after work, listening to music, or reaching out to a loved one, such as a good friend or your support partner (see more on this on page 166). The more you lean into the habit of reflection without judgment, the easier and more productive it will become.

An important part of reflection is gratitude. Gratitude is the felt sense of being thankful for all things in your experience—material possessions, people, pets, food, clean water, electricity, the sunshine on your face, each breath you take. It also means appreciating the challenging experiences, for how you may have grown or learned from them. If we only take the time to focus on what we want but don't have, we'll get stuck in a mindset of negativity. Research shows that the practice of daily gratitude can increase well-being and happiness.[3]

> "It is necessary, then, to cultivate the habit of being grateful for every good thing that comes to you; and to give thanks continuously."
>
> —*Wallace D. Wattles*

Tool #7: Reflection and Gratitude Journal

Journaling reflections about your week and feelings of gratitude is another habit we invite you to practice weekly in the 6-week program.

Whether you'd prefer to use a regular notebook, journal, or your computer, it doesn't matter. I personally love to put physical pen to paper. For me, something about the practice of writing, listing, sometimes even drawing, induces a sense of creativity that makes the whole process more personal and fun. The invitation is to document your experience from the past week. You can customize it however you'd like, but reviewing your action plan by evaluating any successes and barriers for each of your small goals is recommended to fully process and be intentional with your action plan for the next week. Here are some reflection suggestions:

1. *Reflect on events from the past week.* You may want to look at the other tools to jog your memory, such as your refrigerator chart or calendar. Think about conversations you had with your friends or family members, and any other thoughts, emotions, or sensations that come up for you during this exercise. There is no wrong way to journal; simply allowing your thoughts to flow can help you discover things that you might not have been aware of.

2. *Review each small goal in your action plan from the past week.*

   - What were the successes? What were actions or practices that really aligned with your intentions? Celebrate even the small things, like making a salad for dinner or getting out for a walk. The more you acknowledge and identify the little things that worked for you, the more likely it is that they will become long-term habits.

   - What were the barriers? Often when we take the time to evaluate the roadblocks, the answers are right there. Approach these without judgment and take note of what got in the way of achieving your goals. Ask yourself whether any problems you identify are logistical or motivational barriers. For example, if you set a goal to go grocery shopping after work and identified that you did not go because you worked too late or had other events that conflicted with shopping, you might discover that you don't feel motivated to be in a busy grocery store at the end of your workday, and your decision-making may be driven by your desire *not* to go.

- What drives your decisions? The motivation to keep going can be characterized by both internal and external factors. Self-determination theory in psychology says that we are intrinsically motivated to do things that we find to be satisfying and interesting, rather than needing to rely on outside incentives to move us into action.[4] For example, if you're the type of person who wakes up refreshed and ready to go out for a jog in the morning because you crave the runner's high and are awakened by the morning sunshine, that's intrinsic motivation. But if you're like most of the American population that isn't coming close to meeting the recommended physical activity guidelines, you'll likely need something extrinsic such as an engaging fitness class, an appointment with a trainer, or the satisfaction of seeing or feeling the desired changes in your body. So, we recommend reflecting on the decisions you made to act (or not act) on each goal and consider whether you were naturally motivated to follow through or if perhaps you needed a little help. It's okay to be extrinsically motivated. The key is awareness of what you need in order to take action.

3. *Modify or recommit to small goals.* If you find that you are having trouble establishing a routine around a certain goal and you identify through reflecting on the barriers that a motivational problem exists, reflect a little deeper to ask yourself what things will be different in the upcoming week compared to the past week. If you're coming up with the same lack of desire to follow through, it may be time to modify the goal. In the example of not grocery shopping, you might consider whether your motivation to grocery shop could

improve if you move the time you plan to shop, change the method to online grocery delivery, or, if possible, enlist the support of others in your home to lighten the load of this responsibility. This type of honest reflection is where you discover what really needs to change to get past the barrier and begin to build self-trust.

4. *Make a gratitude list.* Start by listing five things you feel grateful for. Try to list five different things each week. Many people do this as a daily practice, but even journaling about what you're thankful for on a weekly basis can be useful. The invitation here is to be easy about it. These don't have to be big things or things directly related to your goals. In fact, remembering to express gratitude for things we may take for granted every day can cultivate a deeper sense of happiness without a perpetual wanting for the next bright, shiny thing to come along, encouraging a more balanced mindset when challenges arise.

"When one door of happiness closes, another opens, but often we look so long at the closed door that we do not see the one that has been opened for us."

—*Helen Keller*

TRUST AND SUPPORT

Trust and support, the final SMART MIND habit for success, forms the foundation for sustained change. When it comes to making behavioral changes, trust begins with self-efficacy. Self-efficacy in psychology is defined as your belief and self-confidence in your ability to achieve and maintain your goals.[5] The theory is that people who have higher levels of inner trust and self-efficacy have an easier time committing to and even getting enjoyment from the behaviors that lead to their goals (that is, building that intrinsic motivation that makes it easier to take action!). Greater self-trust can also help you bounce back more quickly when you get off track and be more self-compassionate and nonjudgmental.

The good news is that self-trust can be cultivated. One way is by celebrating positive behaviors and the changes you've made. This brings awareness to your potential for success and helps foster a mindset that you are capable of making positive changes in your life. As you strengthen self-trust, you can experience even more confidence, resilience, and motivation to keep going.

Another thing that can have a big impact on your self-trust and self-efficacy is defined in psychology by social cognitive theory, which suggests that our behaviors can influence others and are influenced by watching others around us, particularly in social situations, including social media.[6] You can probably think of an example of someone you interacted with socially or saw on social media that made you want to try some new food or product, or visit a particular place.

Research continues to reinforce this theory with health behaviors.[7] A 32-year analysis of more than 12,000 people explored whether weight gain was associated with those in our social circle, such as a spouse, friends, neighbors, and siblings. In this study, a person's chance of becoming obese was predicted to be 57 percent higher if they had a friend who gained excessive weight. Luckily, this has the potential to work in positive ways, too. Those participants who followed weight loss programs that encouraged connection to others for social support were more successful with weight loss than those who did not have a support network. This means that you can increase the likelihood of success with your new habits if you are accountable to others and socialize with healthy, like-minded people. Building trust with a partner provides accountability, motivation, and insight to further strengthen your own inner trust.

Tool #8: Social Support Partner

In the 6-week program, we will ask you to connect with a social support partner beginning in week 1 and then each week after that, so you will want to identify your partner before the program begins. We recommend finding a partner who either has similar goals as yours or has a history of supporting you through challenging times. This person should bring feelings of nonjudgment and make you feel like you are heard and supported. Start by asking this person if they can be available to you once a week to share ideas, discuss challenges, or just hear about your journey.

Beware of recruiting an enabling buddy. Don't choose the friend who you know can easily talk you into going out for happy hour after work instead of going to the gym. If you don't feel like you have the right support partner in your life, there are many online resources where you can build this kind of network. A great website is Meetup.com. Meetup isn't only for health behaviors, but you can narrow your search to your topic of interest and find activities to keep you motivated with your small goals, such as walking groups, fitness challenges, or local community events with campaigns for eating well, exercising, and learning how to cook.

Another option would be to take advantage of some of the wearable technology available today. Apple Watches, Fitbits, and other devices are much more than just step counters. They can do things like track your heart rate zones, monitor different types of exercises (such as weightlifting and stair climbing), and even track your sleep and provide guided breathing sessions for stress management. And probably the best feature: scheduling assistance! Many of them can give you reminders to move at customizable intervals and can deliver messages to do things like pack your lunch before you go to bed or take a midday break for a snack. Automated accountability—now that's a reliable buddy!

CHAPTER 16

Tools for Weight Loss

By Jennifer Ventrelle

We would like to provide some additional tools that are scientifically proven for success in weight loss. If you're interested in the MIND diet specifically for weight loss, you can use these bonus tools to help you with your efforts.

MIND DIET PROGRAM BONUS TOOLBOX FOR WEIGHT LOSS

Bonus Tool #1: Nutrition Tracking App
Bonus Tool #2: Body Weight Scale
Bonus Tool #3: Meal Timing Schedule
Bonus Tool #4: Lifestyle Program or Health Coach

NUTRITION TRACKING APP: A BONUS SELF-MONITORING TOOL

Self-monitoring is a crucial piece of the puzzle when you are trying to lose weight. Research consistently shows a connection between keeping diet records and weight loss.[1] This is one reason we chose Self-Monitoring with the MIND Diet Refrigerator Chart as the first tool in our 6-week program. A closer look at some of this research reveals that how often you keep diet records and how complete the records are matters. One study that followed participants in a diabetes prevention and management program found that the only people who lost a significant amount of weight were the ones who tracked what they ate for an average of 4 or 5 days per week.[2] A review of 59 weight loss studies found that people who tracked all of the foods they ate lost significantly more weight than those who tracked just certain foods (such as the MIND diet's 10 *Foods to Choose* and 5 *Foods to Limit*). This suggests that you'll have more success with weight loss if you're self-monitoring at least 4 days per week and if you track other foods and drinks in addition to the MIND diet foods. We recommend using an app on your smartphone or an online system that can give you some immediate feedback. Some good options include MyNetDiary, Carb Manager, MyFitnessPal, and Lose It. At the very least, a food diary written in a regular notebook can help increase awareness of your eating patterns.

I worked very closely with a client, Tina, whose MIND diet score consistently landed in the top range. She reported feeling more confident in her ability to plan ahead to get in all those brain-healthy leafy greens, other veggies, and whole grains. She was also quite proud of her ability to "stick to" the minimum of 4 sweets each week, as her love for chocolate was one habit at the top of her list of indulgences that sabotaged past weight loss efforts. She was losing weight, but not as quickly as she had hoped. When we discussed the strategies that had helped her with weight loss in the past, she named one prominent tool: self-monitoring.

> "I think I need to start tracking everything I eat. I love the MIND tracker, and even though I'm getting a great score, I wonder if things are slipping through the cracks."
>
> —*Tina B.*

Tina was careful about tracking everything she ate on the refrigerator chart, but when she began using the nutrition tracking app, she noticed that the calories from the foods not counted on the MIND chart began to add up quickly. Some of her favorites were whole-grain crackers and low-fat cheese, which she enjoyed in between meetings, and 2 percent milk, which she loved to have as an evening refreshment. She also noticed that even when her 4 sweets servings turned into a full-on chocolate binge, she still managed to get a therapeutic MIND score by paying closer attention to the list of *Foods to Choose*. This was great news for brain health; however, it was not aligned with her goal of weight loss.

The automated feedback Tina received from the tracking system also allowed her to discover a pattern: she would turn to hearty snacks when feeling stressed from work, and one snack could turn into a mindless eating binge. As soon as Tina realized what was going on, the power was back in her control. She reached her peak weight loss of more than 30 pounds and still returns to her tracking app as a tool when she feels her MINDful eating habits begin to drift.

> "The extra tracker is a tool that has been giving me insight into which things are satisfying or not. Otherwise, I can lie to myself about what my body needs. Thinking back, I can remember rationalizing why I *should* have the extra snack... or eat the chocolate...or order the pizza....I have so much more compassion now for addictions...it's seductive."
>
> —*Tina B.*

BODY WEIGHT SCALE:
A BONUS SELF-MONITORING TOOL

The largest study of long-lasting weight loss results is known as the National Weight Control Registry (NWCR), led by Dr. Rena Wing at Brown Medical School/The Miriam Hospital Weight Control and Diabetes Research Center and Dr. James O. Hill from the University of Colorado.[3] Individuals who had been successful with long-term weight loss of an average of 66 pounds maintained for an average of 5.5 years were followed over time to determine "what's the secret." The first and most referenced behavior was self-monitoring of body weight.

In this study, 75 percent of the participants reported weighing themselves at least once weekly. For weight loss, we believe this is a must for two reasons:

1. *Awareness.* It can be very easy for small fluctuations in weight to turn into large gains — or losses. Neither is good for brain or heart health. We recommend weighing yourself on the same scale on the same day and time each week. It is so simple and takes virtually no time to step on the scale.

2. *Success.* Research shows that the habit of weekly weighing is associated with higher weight loss.[4] And once a week is plenty. Daily weighing may cause you to become overly focused on the number on the scale, which can be a goal but shouldn't be the only focus.

WEIGHT LOSS ON THE MIND?

Self-Monitoring

Tracking intake with the MIND Diet Refrigerator Chart plus a smartphone or online nutrition tracking app can help you identify patterns to aid in weight loss.

Track *all* foods and drinks consumed for 4 or 5 days each week.

Tracking weight patterns with a body weight scale is associated with successful weight loss.

Make a habit to weigh yourself once a week on the same day and time.

SELF-MONITORING AND WEIGHT LOSS TARGETS

You might be wondering what a realistic target could be for weight loss while following the MIND diet. Although the answer to this question will be different for everyone, most healthcare providers recommend starting with weight loss of 5 to 10 percent of initial body weight over 6 to 12 months.[5] One reason is that this level of weight loss can make a significant impact in risk reduction for heart disease, diabetes, and other health complications. Remember, the average weight loss among all participants in the MIND trial was 5.5 percent, aligning with average improvement in cognition for all. We recommend starting with an initial weight loss target of 5 percent of total body weight, with the understanding that you can always set another target after this first one is achieved. Setting small, incremental weight loss targets can be encouraging as you periodically achieve significant milestones, allowing you to stay motivated and even making it feel easier to reach your long-term target.

WEIGHT LOSS ON THE MIND?

Weight Loss Targets

A good weight loss target is 5 to 10 percent of initial body weight over 6 to 12 months.

When it comes to long-term weight loss, the problem is often not that the diets stop working, but that people stop working the diets because they realize that the diets no longer fit into their lifestyle. Here is where your action plan comes into play. It is best to create small goals that you can see yourself building upon to sustain your lifestyle habits over the next 6 to 12 months. It takes a minimum of 6 to 8 weeks to form a habit. So, given the timeline discussed here, if you're gearing up to follow the 6-week program with an added goal of weight loss, you should be open to the idea of following the program beyond the 6 weeks. There will be plenty of ways for you to vary the suggested instructions over the 6 weeks to repeat the program many times in a row with a completely unique experience every time.

MEAL TIMING SCHEDULE: A BONUS MEAL-PLANNING TOOL

We included meal timing specifically as a tool for weight loss, since eating on a regular schedule can prevent excessive hunger, control overall calorie intake, sustain energy levels, and reduce cravings—all good practices for maintaining a healthy weight.

A scientific statement from the American Heart Association (AHA) reviewed recommendations from a variety of studies on meal timing as it relates to cardiovascular disease prevention and weight loss. The purpose of the statement was to produce practical guidelines they call an "Intentional Approach to Eating" for breakfast consumption, eating frequency, and intermittent fasting.[6]

Scheduling Breakfast

The correlation between obesity and skipping breakfast is well known. Seventy-eight percent of the participants in the NWCR reported eating breakfast every day. Research reviewed as part of the AHA's scientific statement suggests that eating early in the day helps you consume less over the course of the day, decreasing the likelihood of overeating. So, the cliché holds true...breakfast really is the most important meal of the day. Here are some common FAQs around the topic of breakfast:

What if I'm not hungry for breakfast?

First, you may be eating too close to bedtime, which could be affecting your hunger signals in the morning. Aim to eat your last meal at least 2 hours before bedtime. If you start eating breakfast, it's likely that you will naturally become hungrier earlier in the day. This is normal; think of it as your body retuning your hunger cues. Pay attention to see if eating earlier reduces your overall intake throughout the day.

What if I don't have time to make breakfast?

Consider some of the "In a Rush" meal ideas from part II that require little prep, such as the Key Lime Smoothie (page 251) or Strawberry Green Breakfast Smoothie (page 252). If you're willing to do a little prep ahead of time, you can make something that will keep well in the freezer and can easily be reheated, such as the Veggie Frittata (page 240) made in a muffin tin.

What if I wake up too late for breakfast?

Don't get too hung up on the traditional context of the idea of "breakfast." In the AHA's report, breakfast was defined as "the first meal of the day that breaks the fast after the longest period of sleep, occurs within 2 to 3 hours of waking, and contains foods and beverages from at least 1 food group." In short, you don't have to eat "breakfast" foods for breakfast.

Can I eat the same breakfast every day?

Research shows that eating the same foods on a daily basis can indeed aid in weight loss.[7] Scheduling a few breakfast ideas that you rotate and eat at the same time each day may be a simple small goal as a part of your action plan that could lead to formation of a long-term habit.

Scheduling Meal and Snack Frequency

The research studies on which the AHA guidelines are based show that consuming frequent meals helps protect the heart and prevent type 2 diabetes. Eating more frequently was associated in some studies with a lower risk for obesity, but other studies showed that eating more frequently coupled with three specific patterns increased the risk for being overweight or obese: (1) when you make unhealthy food choices, (2) when you eat more than six times per day, and (3) when you eat late at night (within 2 hours of bedtime). The habit of late-night eating seems to be the most harmful both for weight status and cardiometabolic risk.[8]

Makes sense, right? If you increase frequency of eating but make poor food choices that are lacking in nutrients or too dense in calories, health risk increases. Likewise, if you're eating too frequently, especially without reducing portions, your calorie intake would increase, and you would actually gain weight. And finally, I think we've all heard that it's not good to eat too late. We may be more likely to overeat due to fatigue and mindless eating; it can interfere with sleep patterns and circadian rhythms, and it may disrupt eating patterns the following day.

A study looking at the relationship between meal timing and weight status suggests the best pattern of meal frequency for maintaining a healthy weight may be three meals and two snacks per day. This was based on the meal patterns of normal weight individuals and those who had successfully lost weight and kept it off.[9] I invite you to think about the times you typically eat meals and snacks to get a better understanding of your current meal-timing pattern. You may want to incorporate scheduling of meals or snacks as a small goal in your action plan to provide more opportunities to incorporate healthy MIND diet foods and optimize your weight loss efforts.

Intermittent Fasting

Intermittent fasting (IF) has become a popular approach for weight loss in recent years. Long-term studies on IF and weight loss are lacking, and researchers don't claim this method to be any more effective than traditional calorie restriction. Furthermore, we don't have any scientific evidence related to the effects of this approach on cognitive decline and dementia.

Some studies have shown IF to be an effective weight loss strategy, producing weight loss of anywhere from 3 to 8 percent of initial body weight over as little as 3 weeks to as long as 6 months.[10] Three different approaches to IF have been studied:

1. Alternate-day fasting, where people consume about 500 calories one day (roughly the equivalent of a small meal or large snack) alternated with a "feast" day in which literally any food and drinks can be consumed in unlimited amounts. So, essentially: starve...binge...starve...binge...repeat.

2. The 5:2 method, where people do 2 fast days and 5 "feast" days per week.

3. Time-restricted eating, where people choose anywhere from 12 to 16 hours as a fasting period only a couple days per week.

A common misconception is that to "intermittent fast" means you should try to go as long as possible without eating. This is not recommended. Anyone who has been on a diet knows how miserable it can be to count the number of hours...minutes...seconds until you're "allowed" to consume the next morsel of food. Glucose is available in the liver to fuel the body in between meals. It takes 10 to 12 hours for all that glucose to be used up. Intermittent fasting works because waiting beyond that amount of time to eat causes a metabolic shift and the body begins to burn fat as the main fuel for energy. The problem comes when hunger levels override your ability to make healthy food choices. So, you could be in a metabolic fat-burning phase after fasting for 16 or more hours, but then overeating puts all that fat right back where you lost it. Additionally, a lifestyle of restricting eating to an 8-hour window or less might get tough when events happen outside this timeframe, such as when you have been invited to someone's home for dinner, are at a social gathering, or are out on a date. So, the question becomes, is fasting a *sustainable* long-term lifestyle change? We don't think things have to be this difficult. Remember that the MIND diet plan is meant to make you feel good!

If you do want to give fasting a try, we recommend beginning with the small goal approach as a part of your action plan. Here are some suggestions:

- *Begin with an overnight fast of 12 hours.* If this works well for you, you may want to expand to 14 hours. Many people try to do the maximum of 16 hours or more, but we do not recommend this. Remember to customize timing for your own schedule — your body may feel better with a wider eating window.

- *Try the time-restricted eating pattern 2 days per week.* Daily fasting may feel like a diet. Studies on people who lost weight with this approach fasted for 1 to 4 days per week. You don't necessarily have to be so prescriptive with an IF regimen. You might try to be a bit more MINDful of your eating times on the weekdays — cutting off eating a bit earlier in the evenings, for example. Then you might find that you can enjoy the flexibility of eating a bit later on the weekends without feeling restricted.

- *Avoid fasting* if you are pregnant or lactating, have a history of disordered eating, have a metabolic disorder such as diabetes, or take medications that can interfere with how your body processes and stores glucose. Intermittent fasting also hasn't been well tested for safety in adults over age 70. If any of these describes you, you may want to avoid or at the very least discuss with your doctor before trying intermittent fasting.

In summary, science seems to support a few key meal-timing guidelines as "an intentional approach to eating" for both brain and heart protection as well as weight loss.

WEIGHT LOSS ON THE MIND?

Meal Timing

Research suggests scheduling mealtimes to be an important weight loss component.

Eat breakfast regularly.

Plan for three balanced meals and one or two snacks daily.

Stop eating 2 hours before bedtime.

Leave 12 to 14 hours between your final meal/snack of the night and your first meal the next day.

We include advice for scheduling mealtimes using the strategies above in week 4 of the 6-week program. For a deep dive into setting up a personalized meal timing schedule and to access an interactive, downloadable meal timing scheduling bonus tool, visit TheOfficial MINDdiet.com.

Scheduling Repeated Meals

If you are used to eating the same or similar types of foods each day, and weight loss is one of your goals, this strategy may help you. Research shows that the more options available at a single meal, the more likely people are to overeat.[11] This makes sense—picture a party with a dessert table filled with plates of cakes, brownies, cookies, etc. Then picture a party with a table with one plate of cookies. Which scenario does the research say causes people to eat more dessert? If you guessed the party with a variety of desserts, that is a good guess! When so many of our taste buds are stimulated, dopamine gets released and the brain's pleasure center gets activated, sending one message: *keep going!*

The theory is that mammals, including humans, have an innate drive to seek out a variety of foods and, therefore, essential nutrients, so as not to starve or become malnourished in times of scarcity. We are far from times of scarcity in our modern developed country. So, after taking a moment to express gratitude for the easily accessible abundance of food, recognize that you can make this brilliant quality of the brain work in our favor. You can try limiting the variety of the foods and drinks that are higher in calories and increasing the variety of foods and beverages that are lower in calories. Eat a variety of vegetables and drink plenty of water or other calorie-free beverages such as sparkling water or tea, for instance. Remember that drinking a full glass of water before each meal and snack is great for weight loss, since water is heavy and takes up a lot of space in the stomach, triggering satiety hormones that tell your brain you're full.

Letting repetition work for you might also include establishing routines in the meal-planning process — for example, having the same type of breakfast or lunch most days or repeating the same dinner by enjoying leftovers once or twice a week. Another strategy would be to target the foods you may have a tendency to overeat, like starches such as rice, potatoes, and pasta. In this case, you could aim to prepare two types of vegetables for a meal and only one type of starch.

Keeping an eye on your MIND Diet Refrigerator Chart can ensure you're eating enough variety for brain and heart health. We recommend repeating two or three of your meals throughout the week. This also makes meal planning much easier and more streamlined.

WEIGHT LOSS ON THE MIND?

Try repeating the same or similar meals throughout the week. Having a variety of vegetables and drinking plenty of water with fewer meal options may assist with weight loss and keep meal planning simple.

LIFESTYLE PROGRAM OR HEALTH COACH: A BONUS TRUST AND SUPPORT TOOL

Some people need a bit more support than having a casual workout partner, program buddy, or high-tech device. If this is true for you, a lifestyle program or personal health coach could be an option through your doctor's office, fitness center, or local community center. It can be very motivating to work with a coach and/or be a part of a group working toward a similar goal.

Let's return once again to the NWCR. Fifty-five percent of the people in this study lost weight with the help of a program. We also know from other important lifestyle intervention and weight loss studies that people who attend programs in groups lose more weight, and that unfortunately, weight is often regained after accountability or support is discontinued.[12] This means that if you're like the majority of people who try to lose weight, you'll likely be more successful with a little help.

All participants in the MIND study worked with a coach weekly for 6 months and then twice monthly for the remaining 2½ years of the study. As mentioned, the average weight loss was 5.5 percent at 6 months, and this average was maintained through the end of the 3-year intervention. They also had opportunities to connect with one another through group sessions, where they shared recipes and tips on how to follow their diets, and exchanged motivational strategies about what kept them moving in the right direction. This can be a great model for your weight loss success!

If you work better one-on-one, I highly recommend making an appointment with a registered dietitian. Many insurance companies cover the cost of wellness visits; or, if you have a condition like obesity, diabetes, or even prediabetes, your doctor might be able to give you a referral. Even if the dietitian you see does not directly take insurance or is out of network with your insurance, they may be able to supply you with a SuperBill, which is essentially a receipt that details the services provided. You can then submit this to your insurance company to seek reimbursement.

You can search for a dietitian in your area through the Academy of Nutrition and Dietetics website at EatRight.org. It's important to work with a professional who has been trained in nutrition, health education, and behavior change counseling. I especially recommend this if your weight loss goal is greater than 5 to 10 percent of your current weight, and it's likely that you'd need more time than 6 weeks. We recommend meeting with your support partner weekly for at least the first 3 months. After 3 months, you can reassess your needs and decide whether you should keep meeting weekly or taper down. As the gaps get wider, more support might be needed. So please, don't be afraid to reach out to your social support partner or group when you need them. Just be sure to view your support person as a coach rather than a crutch. Remember that trust in your own ability is key to building the intrinsic motivation for long-lasting results. You can also visit the website TheOfficialMINDdiet.com for more information or resources for health coaches and the official MIND diet program.

WEIGHT LOSS ON THE MIND?

Successful Weight Loss Maintenance Strategies

Self-monitor weight weekly.

Incorporate breakfast in your meal plan daily.

Join a program or hire a health coach. Meet with them weekly for at least 3 months to build trust and support.

Our goal is to make things simple for you by inviting you to gather the tools you need to get started and then customize your own small changes along the way. You get to decide how structured or fluid you would like to make the program and then monitor what is working for you versus what may need to be altered. Your health coach or other members of your lifestyle program can be a great support in helping you determine these things, but ultimately the final choices are up to you.

> "Excellence-ism is better than perfectionism...you can be excellent at a lot of things, but you don't have to be perfect at anything. And that's an incredible relief!"
>
> —*Tina B.*

CHAPTER 17

Your MINDful Life

by Laura Morris

Now that you are armed with knowledge about the important role diet plays in brain health, let's talk about some other lifestyle habits that may contribute to healthy aging. There is abundant evidence in the scientific literature that in addition to nutrition, other key life-style practices may help your brain perform optimally and preserve cognitive health. These include physical activity, sleep, intellectual and social engagement,[1] and happiness.[2] The exciting news about these practices is that they are greatly within your control. Think of these practices as essential to living a full life of health and longevity.

In each week of the 6-week program, we will give you an opportunity to customize a small goal for yourself. As you read about the habits below, consider whether you may want to incorporate any of them into your program to maximize your MINDful life.

PHYSICAL ACTIVITY

"There is an immediate impact of nutrition and exercise on how well you function, how well you think, how well you feel, and how well your body is working. But there are long-term benefits as well. Exercise and diet are the two primary factors in every chronic disease that starts in middle age: diabetes, heart disease, osteoporosis, you name it."

—*Dr. Martha Clare Morris*

In addition to healthy nutrition, physical activity is one of the best lifestyle practices you can have. Exercise is certainly beneficial to cardiovascular health, and it may provide physical benefits to the brain as well. Exercise promotes neuroplasticity, which is your brain's ability to create new neural connections. This has been specifically found in the hippocampus area of the brain, which is responsible for learning new things. In addition, physical exercise may also be responsible for triggering the release of brain-derived neurotrophic factor (BDNF), one of the key molecules that encourages the growth of new brain cells and is responsible for long-term memory function.[3]

The EXERT trial, led by Dr. Laura Baker, investigated the effects of exercise on brain function in 300 sedentary older adults who already had mild cognitive impairment.[4] The goal was to determine whether a year of moderate-intensity aerobic exercise could prevent cognitive decline or even improve cognition compared to a routine of stretching, balance, and range of motion exercises. Both groups had assistance from trainers at a YMCA. To everyone's surprise, neither group declined in cognitive abilities over the course of 12 months. The authors considered this to be a remarkably positive finding, as it suggests that it's never too late to start an exercise program, even if you are completely sedentary and have mild cognitive impairment. The message is that *consistency* is essential. These individuals preserved their brain function through 30 to 40 minutes of activity, 4 days per week, for a full year—and the type of activity didn't matter! Additionally, the positive effect was found through the help of a support system. This could be a personal trainer but doesn't have to be; a workout buddy can be sufficient. The idea is to have someone who keeps you accountable and shows up for your workouts or even a buddy that checks in with a quick text or phone call.

For healthy individuals without cognitive impairment, we have a framework that tells us how to keep our brains and bodies most fit—or, rather, "FITT." To build an exercise plan curated for your needs, you can refer to the guidelines of the FITT principle, which stands for Frequency, Intensity, Time, and Type. This method helps you design an exercise plan based on factors that are fluid and should be evaluated and modified every 4 to 6 weeks to keep your body and mind challenged.

Frequency represents how often you will be exercising, specifically how many days per week. The Physical Activity Guidelines for Americans, put out by the U.S. Department of Health and Human Services and supported by the American Heart Association, recommends a frequency of 3 to 5 days per week to meet the suggested guidelines. In addition, moderate- to high-intensity strength training should be performed on at least 2 of those days. Bottom line: exercising regularly throughout the week is important for your health and well-being. Deciding how often you will exercise is an important first step to establishing a routine. Just like making changes to your diet, any new exercise program should be incorporated gradually and at a pace that will keep you motivated and not cause burnout or injury. If you're just getting started, 5 days may be too ambitious. Aim to work up to this goal and schedule in your workouts as you would anything else that is important to you.

Intensity refers to the level of difficulty and effort you put into your workout. It ranges from low to high and can make a big difference in the success of your desired results. The easiest way to measure this is by the rate of perceived exertion (RPE). This is an observation of how challenging the exercise is based on a scale of 1 to 10, with 1 being very light and 10 being the highest level of difficulty. The following chart describes the intensity levels from 1 to 10.

Intensity is something to be MINDful of especially if you feel you are not working hard enough or are having difficulty reaching your goals. To maximize benefits, an ideal RPE for aerobic exercise is 6 to 8 and a good goal for strength training is 4 to 6. You may find that a check-in with your RPE will reveal that you could be pushing yourself a bit more. Many people find this method fun and motivating.

RPE SCALE	Exertion signs
1	Very light activity: not engaged in exercise but moving around the house or workplace
2–3	Light activity: could engage in for long periods of time and carry on conversations Example: sustained walk
4–6	Moderate activity: noticeably more challenging, breathing heavy, can hold a short conversation Example: jogging
7–8	Vigorous activity: borderline uncomfortable, short of breath, can speak only in short sentences Example: running
9	Very hard activity: very difficult to maintain exercise intensity, can barely breathe, can speak only a few words Example: running fast or sprinting
10	Maximum effort: can maintain for only a very short time, completely out of breath, unable to talk Example: maximum-effort sprinting

Time refers to the duration of a certain workout or workouts per day. According to the physical activity guidelines mentioned above, that means getting at least 150 minutes—typically 30 minutes 5 days per week—of moderate-intensity aerobic exercise.[5] For those expecting to improve any aspect of their health, such as losing weight or lowering blood pressure, the guidelines say to kick it up to 300 minutes (60 minutes 5 days per week). For example, jogging for 30 minutes or cycling for 60 minutes is the time spent exercising. A good goal is 20 to 60 minutes of continuous or intermittent exercise per workout—although, if all you can fit in is 10 minutes, that is better than nothing! The more you commit time to exercise, the easier it will get to establish a routine.

Type refers to whether the exercise is aerobic or anaerobic. Aerobic exercises are endurance, steady-state exercises that increase a person's heart rate over a sustained period of time, such as jogging or cycling. This type of exercise is great for cardiovascular conditioning and improving muscular endurance. Examples of aerobic exercises are walking, jogging, running, swimming, biking, dancing, rowing, doing the elliptical, stair climbing, and participating in an aerobics class.

Exercises that are anaerobic are weight/strength training (also known as resistance training), sprinting, jumping rope, team sports, mountain biking, high-intensity interval training, and even some yoga and Pilates. You can also do a combination of aerobic and anaerobic exercises, which would be considered interval training.

From team sports to swimming, dancing, cycling, hiking, even mowing the lawn and housework—there are endless ways to exercise. I recommend really leaning into the activities you enjoy or feel you get the most benefit from. If you love lifting weights, then make that the focus of your exercise program. If a runner's high is what you're after, find a running program that fits your schedule. I do recommend that no matter the focus of your program, you still perform a mixture of cardio and strength work to maximize cardiovascular health, gain potential brain health benefits, ensure muscle balance, and prevent injury.

In addition to following the FITT principle, here are some strategies to find the best way to incorporate exercise, enjoyment, and success into your daily routine:

- *Develop an appropriate exercise program for your particular stage of life, body type, and specific health concerns.* Think hard about what you want from an exercise regimen and what time you have to commit to it—this can help you a lot when deciding what your body needs to stay healthy and thrive.

- *Find enjoyable activities.* Are you a social person? Joining a walking group or tennis or pickleball club may be a good option, or even just having a workout buddy to keep yourself accountable. Do you enjoy the outdoors and solitude? Find nature or biking trails near your home to get out and move. If you find you just cannot love any type of exercise, try combining it with something you do enjoy, such as listening to audiobooks or podcasts while you lift weights, or catching up on your favorite TV show while you use the treadmill.

- *Create a habit of movement that works for you.* Think of your habits of physical activity as "exercise" days and "movement" days. The exercise days are the days when you sweat, breathe hard, and try to push beyond what is easy — when you engage in moderate to intense activity. These days should be three to five times per week. The other days of the week are movement days, when you aren't physically pushing yourself with the same intensity. These days are for getting in light to moderate movement, increasing blood flow, and checking in with your muscles. Some examples are taking a brisk walk for 30 minutes, doing yoga or stretches, or enjoying a low-intensity bike ride.

- *Have a growth over goals mindset.* When it comes to goal setting, I like to emphasize growth over goals. What really makes a difference in our daily life and workouts is the growth we can achieve through consistent hard work. Prioritizing your exercise time and focusing on the small steps you take, the 1 percent improvement each day, and the skills you acquire along the way will be the most successful path to achievement. Lay out your workout clothes the night before. Have a set time that's blocked off for exercise to make it a priority every day. Listen to your inner voice and steer self-talk toward a positive view on exercise. Instead of saying "I should work out," say "I *get* to work out" or "I *want* to work out to feel good and energized."

- *Accept changes to your body and adjust as needed.* Almost every person has some ache or pain, musculoskeletal issue, or illness they deal with as they age. It's important to acknowledge these signs and symptoms and meet your body where it is at. If you have an injury or pain in a certain area, take a break from any activity that is exacerbating it. When the pain sub-sides, you can gradually incorporate the activity back in. This does not mean take a break from exercise all together — just the activity that is irritating an injury. A sore knee does not mean you cannot exercise; rather, you can design whole work-outs around other areas of the body, for instance by focusing on upper body weight training and core work until your knee has rested properly. If the pain or discomfort remains after 3 to 6 weeks of rest, make an appointment to see your doctor or an orthopedic specialist, as there could be larger issues that need medical attention.

PHYSICAL ACTIVITY AND WEIGHT LOSS

In the spirit of keeping the 6-week program focused on nutrition, we did not explicitly designate physical activity as a tool for success. However, if you do have a goal of weight loss, we know that it will take more than improved nutrition to sustain your results. Per our national physical-activity guidelines, the amount needed to produce sustained weight loss — 300 minutes — is double the amount needed to maintain general health and well-being.[6]

If you're not at this level, don't get discouraged! The good news is that the intensity of activity does not need to be vigorous to see results. When it comes to physical activity reported by the biggest weight-losers in the National Weight Control Registry, 94 percent increased physical activity mostly by just *walking*.[7] Just remember to pick up the pace a bit. You don't need to be sprinting on the treadmill or sweating bullets in a spin class to see results, but aim for a moder-ate level where you begin to work up a sweat by brisk walking, for example. In this group, 90 percent of the participants exercised an average of 1 hour per day. Okay, this is *a lot* of planned physical activ-ity. If you don't have the time to devote an hour a day, think about elevating the intensity a bit more with a different type of exercise that is more vigorous, such as high-intensity aerobics, a spin class, or jogging if your joints will allow it. Consistency at this level will cut the target back down to 150 minutes, or 30 minutes five times per week.

SLEEP

"Poor sleep quality is a common condition that increases with age, affects the quality of life, and increases the risk of multiple chronic conditions and mortality. High sleep fragmentation was associated with a 50 percent higher risk of developing Alzheimer's disease over 6 years in the Rush Memory and Aging Project, and with a 22 percent increase in the annual rate of cognitive decline."

—*Dr. Martha Clare Morris*[8]

People typically spend about one-third of their lives asleep. There is no question that no matter our age, we all function and think better after a good night's sleep. The National Sleep Foundation recommends that healthy adults get 7 to 9 hours of quality sleep per night.[9] "Sleep disturbance" can be characterized by undesirable sleep duration (fewer than 7 or more than 9 hours per night), poor quality of sleep, or inability to fall or remain asleep due to conditions such as insomnia or sleep apnea. Research shows that these types of sleep disturbances are associated with a higher risk for Alzheimer's disease as well as a greater risk for inflammation and cardiovascular disease.[10] Pay attention to any signs of trouble sleeping at night, irregular sleep/wake patterns, daytime sleepiness, loud snoring, problems breathing during sleep, or any unusual behaviors at night in you or your partner if you have one—these could indicate a sleep disturbance, and you should consult your doctor for guidance.

So many factors can cause sleep disturbance—stress, illness, poor diet, physical inactivity, burden from work and family responsibilities—many of which are within our realm of control. If you think you may be experiencing a sleep disturbance, here are simple guidelines you might consider customizing into small goals as a part of your action plan at some point during the 6-week program:

- *Create a bedtime routine.* Wake up and go to bed around the same time each day, even on weekends. This can help set your body's natural clock (circadian rhythms) to ensure you do not oversleep, thereby impacting your ability to fall asleep the next night. Pay attention to when your body is getting sleepy. Set up a routine for yourself that tells your body it is time to sleep — for example, take a warm shower or bath, read, drink herbal tea, or engage in meditation or prayer. Additionally, try to avoid looking at the clock during the night or intentionally setting alarms earlier than needed to wake up.

- *Create a restful sleep environment.* You want your bedroom to be a peaceful, calm space — so keep it cool, dark, and quiet. Limit items that may trigger your brain to be stimulated, such as cell phones, computers, TV, or clutter. You'll also want to keep the bed for sleeping and other adult activities only.

- *Limit the amount of caffeine and alcohol you consume.* Caffeine is a stimulant that can impact the onset of sleep and reduce sleep time, efficiency, and quality. The half-life of caffeine is 4 to 6 hours, which means that it takes double this time to completely clear caffeine from the body. Consuming caffeine in the afternoon or evening can block the sleep-promoting chemical called adenosine in our brain. Similarly, drinking alcohol has been linked to poor sleep quality and duration, particularly interfering with REM (rapid eye movement) sleep, the phase when much of the restoring and repair work is done in the body. With this in mind, avoid drinking alcohol less than 4 hours before bedtime to reduce the risk of sleep disruptions.

- *Refrain from electronics 30 minutes before bedtime.* The light emitted from your electronics interferes with your circadian rhythms and melatonin production in the brain. Light and darkness tell us when to feel awake or sleepy. Basically, all the blue light from your cell phone, tablet, computer, clock, and TV is sending light into your brain, telling you it is daytime.

- *Consider the connection between sleep and weight loss.* If you're having trouble losing weight, you may want to investigate your sleep habits. This could be as simple as tracking your sleep hours or any disturbances in your journal. You could follow every recommendation in this book to a T, but if your sleep patterns are disrupted and hormones are imbalanced, your ability to lose weight could be impaired. For those looking to lose weight, this would be a great nominee for a small goal in the 6-week program if sleep is something that you feel you could improve.

INTELLECTUAL AND SOCIAL ENGAGEMENT

"Social structure is one of the primary areas that has been pretty consistent from one study to the next. People who are more socially active and engaged and have good interactions in social situations are protected from developing clinical Alzheimer's disease. There are all these synaptic connections in the brain that are generated through cognitive activities. The more synaptic connections there are, the more neural connections there are that can weave themselves around any kind of pathologies that develop in the brain. That's the theory of cognitive reserve. The more you challenge yourself and stimulate the brain, the more connections you'll have, and therefore more cognitive reserve. Learning a new instrument or a new language, engaging in social activities, forming new relationships, all of those things help to build this cognitive reserve."

—*Dr. Martha Clare Morris*

191

Social Connection

Social contact increases cognitive reserve and encourages health behaviors through the power of health networks.[11] In contrast, research shows that social isolation increases risk for dementia. These findings have been consistent across cultures; a 10-year study of Japanese older adults identified five areas through which to maximize social connections, including marital interactions, mutual support from family members, connection with friends, community group participation, and being involved in paid work.[12]

Positive social relationships support the well-being of everyone involved and encourage all parties to communicate respectfully and promote a feeling of acceptance. Bottom line: the way in which we interact with people matters.

You know the saying, "Treat others the way you want to be treated"? It is amazing how well this can be reciprocated. It could benefit you to consider ways to incorporate social engagement into a small goal as a part of your action plan throughout the 6-week program. Here are some simple guidelines for fostering positive social connections:

- *Be a good listener.* My mom always said most people just want to be heard. Really listen to what someone is telling you and let them know you hear what they are saying. This shows that you are interested and understand what they are saying.

- *Provide affirmation and show empathy.* Acknowledging and relating to another person's feelings without judgment is one of the best ways to build connections. This validates the other person's feelings and builds trust.

- *Accept and celebrate differences.* We are all vastly different from one another and have had diverse life experiences, so expecting people to react or think the same way is not reasonable. Be appreciative of varying perspectives and accept that they are not right or wrong—just different.

- *Be present.* Put away cell phones, electronics, and even your to-do list. Be with someone and experience the moment with them without distractions or outside pressures. Value that uninterrupted time to truly make a connection.

- *Learn to trust.* Trust is the foundation of any close relationship. It is crucial to our ability to be fully transparent and vulnerable. It allows us to be open not only to receiving feedback from friends and family, but also to giving it.

- *Avoid gossip.* It's hard to trust someone who gossips. After all, if they can talk about someone else, it's easy to assume that they can talk about you. Unless you are truly trying to help someone, gossip has no benefit to you or your friends.

- *Choose people who make you feel good about yourself.* Socializing is a time for laughing, sharing, and feeling joy. Connect with folks who want this same experience and hold on tight to these relationships.

"They may forget what you said—but they will never forget how you made them feel."

—*Carl Buehner*

Challenging Your Brain with New Learning

In the world of Alzheimer's research, research shows that a large number of people have significant plaques and tangles in their brain, yet they never clinically manifest the disease.[13] Their cognitive abilities remain intact up until their death. The main theory for why this happens is that these individuals had an abundance of neurons and synaptic connections, otherwise known as neural reserve, to complete a thought, task, movement, etc., even with those plaques and tangles. This is exciting because it suggests that building this reserve is protective against actual disease, and that we can stimulate the brain to develop these neural pathways. The benefits of challenging your brain in this way include improvement in memory, speed of thinking, finding words, and capacity to listen.

Here are some ideas for challenging yourself cognitively, which you might consider incorporating as part of your action plan in one of your small goals in the 6-week program:

- *Learn a new skill.* This is a fun way to really challenge yourself. When you look at kids, you see how they're learning new skills at every turn. Approach new activities like a child — by being completely open to the experience. Love food? Take a cooking class. Always been interested in learning guitar? Sign up for private lessons. You will be surprised by the variety of activities and skillsets that are available to you.

- *Choose active over passive entertainment.* Sometimes we just want to plop in front of the TV after a long day. This is fine to do every once in a while, but try not to make it the norm. Instead, seek out mentally stimulating forms of entertainment. Try playing board games or cards. Or grab a great book and learn about something new.

- *Make learning and socializing part of your routine.* If you are learning a new skill, set up a schedule to make it a part of your routine. Make weekly dates or meet up with friends. Aim to be social at least twice a week.

HAPPINESS

"There have been studies in the Alzheimer's field that have shown anxiety and negative stress put you at greater risk of dementia. There have also been studies that have looked at people who have a purpose in life and a positive outlook, and these individuals are less likely to develop Alzheimer's disease. There does seem to be something around that emotional psychological component that is protective of Alzheimer's disease."

—*Dr. Martha Clare Morris*

Psychological health and happiness, including optimism and a sense of purpose in life, has been named by the American Heart Association as a foundation for cardiovascular health.[14] In contrast, we know that negative mind-states such as mental stress, anxiety, and depression can increase risk for cardiovascular disease and dementia.[15]

Optimism

The way we view the world can influence our mental and physical health—along with how we age. It can be hard in the information age to maintain a positive outlook about the world, especially when we hear about every tragedy the minute it happens. Here are some strategies to consider customizing as a part of your 6-week program action planning:

- *Accept adversity.* Life is full of obstacles and heartbreak, but the more we accept them as a part of life and look for the teachable moments, the easier it will be to move forward and focus on the positive things.

- *Give to others.* My grandmother always said if you are feeling down, give something to someone else. This could be as easy as a note to someone appreciating who they are, or maybe flowers or a book. Feeling overwhelmed by the state of the world? Donate your time or money to a cause that is meaningful to you. Action is one of the best ways to bring hope.

- *Reduce the amount of noise and news going into your brain.* Try minimizing these exposures by checking the news only once per day and limiting social media that may induce negative thoughts and feelings. Turn off notifications that may be overwhelming your brain with negative information.

- *Try positive thinking.* Positive thinking isn't about ignoring hard or tragic situations. It is okay to feel angry, sad, or distressed. Shifting your self-talk to a more positive and encouraging tone can influence your ability to regulate your behavior, feelings, and thoughts under stress. If you need reassurance or validation from others, try giving it to yourself first.

- *Practice gratitude.* Journaling, writing letters, or even just saying out loud what you are grateful for has been shown to reduce stress, improve self-esteem, and build resilience in difficult times. Start and end your day with expressing this gratitude. Throughout the 6-week program, we will encourage this practice to help build this habit.

Living Life with Purpose

Having a sense that who you are, what you do in the world, and how you contribute to the things you care about are indications that you are living a life with purpose. Having a sense of purpose in life has been associated with better overall cognition, memory, and executive functioning.[16]

In times of uncertainty or stress, it can be challenging to fully live a life with purpose. Here are some strategies to consider customizing for small goals:

- *Surround yourself with people who inspire you.* Being around people who make a difference in the world and inspire you to make positive change can influence your own actions. Seek out people who motivate you in a positive way.

- *Explore your interests.* Are there topics you frequently bring up or post about on social media? These are good indicators of things that may bring purpose into your life. Seek out education and community around these topics.

- *Think about issues that concern you and find ways to help.* One of the best ways to feel empowered is to get involved in a cause that is deeply rooted in your beliefs. Is climate change on your mind and causing anxiety? Join one of the many online clubs or organizations that have tips, tricks, and ways to donate your time and money to make a difference.

"The purpose of life...is to live it, to taste experience to the utmost, to reach out eagerly and without fear for newer and richer experience."

—*Eleanor Roosevelt*

We like to think that all of these lifestyle factors are much like the neural pathways in the brain. The more pathways you create for yourself—by adopting various lifestyle habits—the better your chances of living a long and disease-free life. Nutrition, physical activity, sleep, intellectual and social engagement, and happiness are all within your control and can have tremendous implications for your MINDful life.

PART IV

THE OFFICIAL MIND DIET 6-WEEK PROGRAM

By Laura Morris and Jennifer Ventrelle

"Challenge yourself: it's the only way you will get better."
—*Dr. Martha Clare Morris*

CHAPTER 18

6 Weeks to a Healthy MIND

Hooray, we have made it to the program! Now that you have an arsenal of tools in your back pocket, it is time to start the Official MIND Diet 6-Week Program. For an overview of the entire 6-week program, refer to the appendix of this book to easily follow along.

To set the foundation for sustainable lifestyle change, we have built the program around the five SMART MIND habits (Self-Monitoring, Meal Planning, Action Planning, Reflection, and Trust and Support) during each of the 6 weeks. See the diagram on the following page for a visual of how the habits build on one another and the cycle repeats each week. This will help keep you in the flow of the program.

The SMART MIND habit cycle begins with Self-Monitoring using the MIND Diet Refrigerator Chart so that you can get an idea of your current eating habits and how you'll want to adapt them. Then you'll move onto Meal Planning, with a variety of tools for time management and prioritizing the activities required for healthy eating. Information from the self-monitoring and meal-planning habits will help you customize the weekly Action Plan, made up of two suggested small goals plus an optional third small goal of your choice. Toward the end of the week, you'll record your MIND diet score in a journal, and be encouraged to do some Reflection on your action plan so you can celebrate successes, highlight improvements that could be made for the following week, and foster MINDful gratitude and self-trust. You'll continue to build Trust and Support by

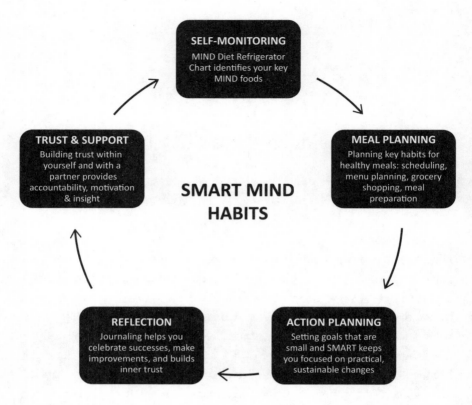

connecting with a social support partner to increase accountability and motivation, as well as to gain insight into which pieces of the lifestyle plan are working well or might need a shift. The following week, the process begins again with Self-Monitoring, with a fresh MIND Diet Refrigerator Chart and MIND Diet Score.

WEEK 1: YOUR BASELINE MIND SCORE AND MEAL PLAN

Welcome to week 1! This week is all about seeing what your current MIND Diet Score is and getting comfortable with meal planning. This is a week to get in touch with the planner in you—whatever your style may be, without judgment. Focus on figuring out what does and does not work for you and your family.

Week 1 Self-Monitoring: Using the MIND Diet Refrigerator Chart on page 136, track all MIND diet foods—both *Foods to Choose* and *Foods to Limit*—without changing your eating habits. You will focus on serving sizes of each food and how often you are consuming these foods. Filling out the chart by tallying your foods soon after you eat them is the best way to ensure that you won't forget what you've eaten. If you don't think it's feasible to keep the chart handy or if this feels overwhelming, we suggest finding a time at the end of the day—for example, just before bedtime—to fill it out. At the end of the week, add up your points to determine your first weekly MIND Diet Score. This score may be different from your score on the MIND Diet Quiz on page 51 that asked about your intake over the past year, since the current method is based on your actual intake versus your recall of how often you ate each of the foods over a whole year with the quiz. Be sure to save your completed charts at the end of each week, because we will be reflecting on them in week 6.

Week 1 Meal Planning: As discussed, we will ask you to begin to build your meal-planning skills by scheduling the meal-planning activities. Below are steps for establishing a template for your meal plan using a Calendar with Reminders:

CALENDAR WITH REMINDERS

INSTRUCTIONS:

1. Choose a calendar that has weekly and monthly views with reminders.
2. Fill in your existing events and obligations.
3. Add new habits of menu planning, grocery shopping, and meal preparation on the same days/times each week for 1 month.
4. Look for conflicts between your existing events and new habits and make a choice to prioritize or move items accordingly as events or personal intentions shift.

Once you have your calendar set up with menu planning, grocery shopping, and meal prepping for the month, focus on just the current week. Using your calendar, begin to fill in your menu by writing in one meal per day for the week. We recommend beginning with dinners. This includes dinners you prepare at home, restaurant meals, leftovers, etc. Again, you are not changing anything this week, just getting into the habit of meal planning. So, if you are not currently in the habit, you can get a feel for what this would be like by thinking back to meals you had the previous week; or if you eat dinner out 5 nights a week, write down the restaurants/food delivery that you will have each night. Likewise, if you're not currently in a grocery-shopping and meal-prepping routine, simply begin by creating space in your daily life to accommodate these activities. Perhaps you go grocery shopping sporadically and only meal prep some of the time. This week, become familiar with your baseline habits and consider what it would be like to do these activities weekly on the days/times that you've chosen.

WEEK 1 ACTION PLAN

Small Goal #1: Track all MIND diet foods without changing eating habits. Tally your MIND points at the end of the week for each food and record your MIND Diet Score in your journal.

Small Goal #2: Schedule one menu item each day without changing eating habits.

Week 1 Action Planning: Since everyone will be at different skill levels when starting this program, we are offering two small goals that can be customized. For example, if planning a meal every day feels overwhelming, you may want to customize the goal to plan one meal per day for just 4 days this week. Alternatively, if you are already accustomed to planning meals, you may want to add a third goal to schedule a new recipe into your menu.

Refer to page 160 if you need a refresher on how to make sure your small goals are SMART. We also recommend posting your action plan somewhere visible to keep the goals at the forefront of your mind.

Week 1 Reflection: This is where you'll determine what you're ready (or not ready) to do. Reflecting on your week and each of the small goals in your action plan will give you great insight for week 2. You can use the following exercise as a template for your reflection and gratitude journaling each week:

REFLECTION AND GRATITUDE JOURNAL

INSTRUCTIONS:

1. Reflect on events from the past week.
2. Review your action plan, evaluating successes, barriers, and your decision-making for each small goal.
3. Modify or recommit to small goals.
4. List 5 new things for which you feel grateful.

What was your MIND Diet Score?

What was your experience with establishing a meal planning routine?

What successes or barriers came up around planning one menu item per day?

Since week 1 is largely focused on establishing a baseline for where you are with your MIND Diet Score and meal planning activities, it's a nice reminder to bring an attitude of nonjudging to your reflection journaling. You're not in competition with anyone but yourself—evaluate your MIND chart and your ability to plan one menu item daily by pointing out what worked well for you and noting areas for improvement. If something feels unrealistic, you can modify the goal or make the decision to recommit to the goal until you're ready to move onto week 2.

Don't forget to conclude your weekly reflection with a gratitude list. Even small things you are grateful for help cultivate feelings of positivity and happiness. You may be fortunate enough to have the basic skills to read the words on this page, the capabilities to absorb and recall the information later, the means to access nourishing food, the ability to prepare your own food, and the determination to play an active role in your own health.

Week 1 Trust and Support: To lay the foundation for trust and support, we recommend identifying a consistent time each week to meet with your social support partner. Plan to have some type of weekly contact with your partner for at least the 6 weeks of the program. You might check in by phone every Sunday or Monday at 10 a.m. or take a midweek afternoon or evening walk to go over your small goals or areas you might be getting stuck. Remember that the best way to form a habit is to practice it on the same day and at the same time each week, so establishing a reliable schedule for you and your support partner will be helpful in implementing this habit.

WEEK 1 WEIGHT LOSS ON THE MIND

BONUS TOOLS FOR WEIGHT LOSS:

Nutrition Tracking App

Body Weight Scale

Calculate your 5% weight loss goal and record it in your journal. Establish a habit to weigh yourself weekly at the same day and time each week.

If you're aiming for weight loss, there are a couple of additional tools recommended for week 1. It's a good idea to track your food intake using a nutrition tracking app such as one of the options mentioned on page 169, in addition to the refrigerator chart. Most of these apps do the calculations for you once you answer questions about your height, weight, age, gender, activity level, and goals for weight loss. Start the first week without changing habits, even though the system may let you know that you may not be meeting the recommended targets. Remember that you're trying to get a baseline idea of where your habits are before changing anything.

This is also true for body weight. To consider week 1 your baseline or initial weight, you will need a body weight scale so you can get into the routine of weighing yourself on the same day and at the same time each week. Your weight can be recorded in your nutrition tracking app or kept in your journal.

You should also get a sense for what a realistic weight goal would be. You can add this to your journal as a long-term goal. As you may recall, most medical practitioners recommend a target of 5 to 10 percent of initial body weight over 6 to 12 months. For this program, we recommend having an initial goal set at 5 percent and repeating the program in its entirety or noting the key components you believe contributed to your weight loss success along the way until you achieve that goal. To calculate your 5 percent goal, multiply your current weight by 0.05. You can then subtract this from your baseline weight to determine your long-term weight goal. When this is achieved, you can reevaluate a new long-term goal as many times needed to achieve a healthy weight.

WEEK 2: LEAFY GREENS, OTHER VEGETABLES, AND BERRIES

Welcome to week 2! This week is all about a variety of vegetables and one important fruit, while introducing you to the process of meal planning with the MIND foods. You'll focus on the leafy green vegetables, other vegetables, and berries. In addition to focusing on consuming a MIND-healthy dose of these colorful foods, you will also aim to reduce your *Foods to Limit* from what they were last week (if needed).

Week 2 Self-Monitoring: This is the week we start to adjust and make changes to keep track of the MIND diet points for leafy green vegetables, other vegetables, berries, and the MIND diet *Foods to Limit* using the refrigerator chart. Although we recommend target servings for optimal brain health, the most important part for your individual plan is that you improve from baseline. So, if your baseline MIND chart from last week shows 0 servings of leafy greens, then maybe 3 servings per week would be a realistic target for you. The same goes for your *Foods to Limit*. If you currently eat 10 servings of red and processed meats per week, a more realistic target could be 5 servings per week. Focus on improving and cementing your habits around these foods.

Here are your *Foods to Choose* targets for this week:

Vegetables and Fruit	MIND Food Points	
Leafy Green Vegetables (LG) **Goal:** 1 serving/day **Serving size:** 1 cup raw or ½ cup cooked	0–2 servings/week	0
	3–6 servings/week	0.5
	7+ servings/week	1
Other Vegetables (OV) **Goal:** 1 serving/day **Serving size:** ½ cup, cooked or raw	0–4 servings/week	0
	5–6 servings/week	0.5
	7+ servings/week	1
Berries (Ber) **Goal:** 5 servings/week **Serving size:** ½ cup	0 servings/week	0
	1–4 servings/week	0.5
	5+ servings/week	1

Here are your *Foods to Limit* targets that you will track through the end of the program:

Saturated Fats	MIND Food Points	
Red & Processed Meats (RM) **Goal:** 0–3 servings/week **Serving size:** 3–5 ounces	0–3 servings/week	1
	4–6 servings/week	0.5
	7+ servings/week	0
Butter & Stick Margarine (But) **Goal:** 0–1 serving/day **Serving size:** 1 teaspoon	0–7 servings/week	1
	8–13 servings/week	0.5
	14+ servings/week	0

Full-Fat Cheese (Chs) **Goal:** 0–2 servings/week **Serving size:** 1 ounce		0–2 servings/week	1
		3–6 servings/week	0.5
		7+ servings/week	0
Fried Foods (Fri) **Goal:** 0–1 serving/week **Serving size:** 1 serving		0–1 serving/week	1
		2–3 servings/week	0.5
		4+ servings/week	0
Sweets, Pastries & Sweet **Drinks (Swt)** **Goal:** 0–4 servings/week **Serving size:** 1 treat or 8-ounce drink		0–4 servings/week	1
		5–6 servings/week	0.5
		7+ servings/week	0

To really focus on the small changes, we recommend that you track only these three categories from the *Foods to Choose* list this week, plus the *Foods to Limit*. We will take this approach with different foods over the next 4 weeks so that you can fully explore the different MIND foods and take your time developing the habit of meal planning. Remember to keep your chart somewhere safe so you can do the reflection exercise in week 6.

Week 2 Meal Planning: Start by taking a look at your calendar for the upcoming week. If the day/time that you chose for scheduling your menu items last week worked well, you may want to set it as a regular time. Last week, the goal was not to change anything, but simply to get into the habit of meal planning. This week, you can take the same approach with the added intention of integrating more vegetables and berries into the routine. Now is the time to plan out when and at which meals you will be eating your leafy greens, other veggies, and berries.

Here are some examples of how to plan for these MIND foods. Look at your calendar for the week and pick one meal a day where you will have either a leafy green salad, a green smoothie, or cooked greens as a menu item. Do the same for the other vegetable serving you are aiming to get daily. The last thing you will do on your calendar is plan out when you will eat your berries. Once you have scheduled this week's MIND foods, finish planning the rest of your meals for the week. This could mean filling in the whole week or just sticking to dinners, whatever makes sense for you.

Next, write out your grocery list and shop accordingly for the week ahead. Consider whether your planned day/time of the week is still possible or change to a better time for the week. If possible, you'll want to pick a day of the week that you can stick to most of the time. If your schedule is dynamic or you feel too busy to get to the grocery store each week, food delivery systems such as Instacart or Amazon Fresh can be good options; they can save you time and potentially even money through discount codes and by helping you avoid impulse purchases. There are also companies like Imperfect Foods (ImperfectFoods.com) and Misfits Market (MisfitsMarket.com) that buy up "imperfect" items that would otherwise go to waste, in addition to overstock/surplus organics and food items at a discounted price.

Week 2 Action Planning: Before committing to the action plan, check to see if any of the small goals need customizing by making them SMART. For example, if you scored 0 for each of the leafy greens, other veggies, and berries on your refrigerator chart last week, you may want to make small goal #1 more realistic by focusing on just leafy greens instead of all three MIND foods this week. Or, if you are already in the habit of planning menus with full meals, you can continue to track all 10 *Foods to Choose* and then get a new MIND diet score at the end of the week. If you're feeling confident about your two small goals, this could be a week to consider adding a third goal to your action plan in the area of physical activity, sleep, or one of the other habits you believe could be improved to optimize your brain health. Revisit chapter 17 for a review of the other brain-healthy MINDful life habits.

Week 2 Reflection: Week 2 will be a time to examine your intake of *Foods to Limit* and think about the environment you are in when you overindulge in these foods.

What did you notice about your intake of the *Foods to Limit* this week? Do you eat more fried food when out socializing at a restaurant? Do you eat a lot of sweets at night before bed? Are you snacking on chips in the car during an afternoon commute? Start to become

---

WEEK 2 ACTION PLAN

Small Goal #1: Track leafy green vegetables, other vegetables, berries, and the 5 *Foods to Limit*. Tally your MIND points at the end of the week and check it with the MIND targets for each tracked food.

Small Goal #2: Schedule leafy green vegetables, other vegetables, and berries into your menu. Make a grocery list and go shopping on your scheduled day to be prepared to incorporate these foods into your routine.

---

aware of your surroundings and situations when consuming the *Foods to Limit*. Begin to think of alternatives that may help you stay on track. This could mean eating a salad with protein before you go out with friends so you don't overindulge with restaurant food. Or it could mean switching to a cup of herbal tea and some berries or other fruit instead of sugary treats in the evening. You could also prepare to-go containers of popcorn and nuts for a car ride in place of chips.

How sustainable do the meal planning activities of scheduling menu items and grocery shopping feel? This week you will also continue to reflect on successes and barriers that can inform the upcoming week. Check in to see if the behaviors you're setting up feel sustainable. If you have scheduled a day/time to do menu planning and grocery shopping, ask yourself how this feels among the other activities in your regular routine. Could these new activities be incorporated regularly every week?

Conclude your journal reflection entry for the week with a few new things for which you feel grateful in this moment.

Week 2 Trust and Support: You will want to continue to meet with your social support partner this week, so check in to see if the day/time you've established feels right for both of you. If you're finding this has become cumbersome, identify ways to make it easier—for instance, by cutting meetings shorter or switching to a video or phone call. The check-in should be supportive enough to allow you to share your experiences throughout the week and exchange feedback, but not a burden that hinders your progress. It's important to find a healthy balance here.

WEEK 2 WEIGHT LOSS ON THE MIND

BONUS TOOLS FOR WEIGHT LOSS:

Nutrition Tracking App

Body Weight Scale

Self-monitoring all food and drinks by using a nutrition tracking app can help with your weight loss efforts.

Use a body weight scale to weigh yourself once weekly to remain focused on a holistic approach to healthy habit changes.

As mentioned in chapter 16, research shows that people who self-monitor all foods, rather than just a subset of foods, may be more successful with weight loss. So, if your goal is to lose weight, you may have already begun using a nutrition tracking app as a bonus tool to self-monitor more than just the MIND foods. If using a nutrition tracking app seems overwhelming to you, you may just want to continue tracking with the refrigerator chart, but be sure to continue tracking *all* the MIND foods as you did in week 1. Self-monitoring all the foods each week of the program could give you an advantage when it comes to weight loss.

We also encourage continued tracking of your weight each week and logging it in your journal. We don't recommend weighing yourself more than once weekly. Our bodies have fluid shifts that can cause weight to fluctuate from day to day. It's best to limit weighing to once weekly to avoid becoming overly focused on the number. Also, remember to be patient with yourself. Sustainable habits take time to develop.

WEEK 3: UNSATURATED FATS — EVOO AND NUTS

Welcome to week 3! This week is all about taking in a brain-healthy dose of unsaturated fats from plants—EVOO and nuts, including nut butters and seeds. In addition, you will continue to aim for a healthy range of the foods to limit. This week is also an opportunity to experiment with new recipes.

Week 3 Self-Monitoring: This week, you'll track EVOO and nuts plus the MIND diet *Foods to Limit* using the MIND Diet Refrigerator Chart.

In addition to continuing to track the 5 *Foods to Limit*, here are your targets for this week:

Unsaturated Fats	MIND Food Points	
Extra-Virgin Olive Oil (EVOO) **Goal:** 2 servings/day **Serving size:** 1 tablespoon	0–6 servings/week	0
	7–13 servings/week	0.5
	14+ servings/week	1
Nuts & Seeds (Nut) **Goal:** 5 servings/week **Serving size:** 1 ounce nuts or seeds or 2 tablespoons nut/seed butter	0 servings/week	0
	1–4 servings/week	0.5
	5+ servings/week	1

You may be wondering about your MIND foods from last week and whether you should keep tracking those as well. This is entirely up to you. If you already had a good base intake of those foods and did well with them, you can keep tracking the leafy greens, other vegetables, and berries this week along with the new MIND foods. If you feel like you need to keep things simple, focus only on EVOO and nuts. At the end of the week, store or save week 3's chart with the ones from weeks 1 and 2.

Week 3 Meal Planning: Here is the time to plan your intake of EVOO and nuts. This week while scheduling your menu items, you can schedule in these MIND foods and start looking for recipes or new ways to incorporate them. This may be easier than you think.

Planning healthy meals is all about layering food with delicious and nutritious ingredients, especially when it comes to these fantastic fats. If you've been focused on planning for one meal such as dinner up until now, this is a good time to start identifying regular routine meals for breakfast and/or lunch that are healthy and work for your schedule. The more consistent and predictable these meals are, the easier it will be to plan for them. You can look for recipes in part V or refer back to part II for some "In a Routine" or "In a Rush" ideas for breakfasts and lunches (specifically chapter 9 for EVOO and nuts).

Whether you add menu items for breakfast and/or lunch or just stick with dinners for the week, consider recipes that could help build out the menu. Adding recipes may also help you include last week's MIND foods of leafy greens, other veggies, and berries in your menu planning, even if you're not tracking those this week. You can still be MINDful of getting these foods in when you can without specifically scheduling them in your menu. After you've planned your menu, make your grocery list and shop for your foods on your designated shopping day.

Week 3 Action Planning:

WEEK 3 ACTION PLAN

Small Goal #1: Track EVOO and nuts, plus the *Foods to Limit*. Tally your MIND points at the end of the week and check with the MIND target for each tracked food.

Small Goal #2: Schedule EVOO and nuts into your menu. Consider recipes that could help build your weekly menu. Make a grocery list and go shopping on your scheduled day to prepare to incorporate these foods into your routine.

Week 3 Reflection: In week 3 you will reflect on **how your eating cues and hydration may be influencing the quality of your food choices.** It can be common to reach for unhealthy choices such as fried foods and high-fat/high-sugar foods when your basic needs are not met. When you adequately nourish and hydrate your body, you are less likely to crave these unhealthy foods. Are you skipping meals and often finding yourself ravenously hungry? Are you eating balanced meals of vegetables, protein, carbohydrates, and fats to satiate your energy needs? Are you drinking enough water or are you dehydrated? Skipping meals or eating unbalanced meals can send your brain demands for instant calories from sugar and fats, and dehydration can mask as hunger, causing you to overeat.

It's also good to **determine what motivates you to eat.** Check in to see if you may be eating for reasons other than true hunger, such as when you're feeling difficult emotions, when you're feeling tired or distracted by watching TV or working on the computer, or when you're bored. Reflect by examining the times you may have overindulged on the *Foods to Limit* and what triggers may have contributed. For example, do you have trouble keeping portions of these foods to a reasonable size? If you see a bowl of potato chips, is it hard to control yourself from eating the whole bowl? Remember that this has to do with activation of the "pleasure centers" in the brain, which can *temporarily* reward you with good feelings, causing you to eat more.

Often, the *Foods to Limit* are eaten out of habit, not necessarily hunger. Start to reflect on swaps you could make or activities you could pursue to change up these triggers to overindulge. If you find that you eat when bored, try keeping books scattered around your home to pick up and read instead of snacking, or, better yet, call a friend for a catch-up. If you want to keep your hands busy during TV time, try playing solitaire or knitting during your show. Or if you do need a snack, plan a healthy option and portion it out.

Another strategy is to engage in non-food-related activities that can activate those pleasure centers and make you feel good, such as listening to music, exercising, helping others, or even seeking help or positive feedback from others.

Begin to identify any triggers for eating that could be modified into healthier habits. For instance, you might need to pack a few healthy snacks and a reusable water bottle to have on hand during your busy day to avoid getting overly hungry and dehydrated. Another strategy could be to rate your hunger level on a scale of 1 to 10 before eating to bring awareness to your hunger cues and any urge to eat in the absence of hunger.

Week 3 Trust and Support: Keep up the momentum with your social support partner. Consider making this fun by exploring some type of challenge or another way to get motivated. This could mean a friendly competition with your partner based on the MIND targets or joining a wellness competition online or in your community. The YMCA has a lot of local programming, and a fantastic resource for seniors is the Alzheimer's Association, which has social and community resources for those living with dementia, caretakers of those with dementia, and even healthy individuals looking to support the cause and keep their minds and bodies in shape. There are locations all over the United States; check for your local chapter at alz.org. Review chapter 15 for more ideas to enhance support.

WEEK 3 WEIGHT LOSS ON THE MIND

BONUS TOOLS FOR WEIGHT LOSS:

Nutrition Tracking App

Body Weight Scale

Continue to track weight weekly and record in your journal.

Take inventory this week of the most helpful tools. Celebrate the successes and be kind to yourself when unpacking barriers.

As usual, if you're aiming for weight loss, check in with your weekly weight and record it in your journal. This is a good week to decide what the most helpful tools have been and what you could let go of for now. For example, if you're attempting to track all the MIND foods or you've chosen to use a nutrition tracking app along with the MIND tracker, and you find yourself overwhelmed, consider using the refrigerator chart to track only the designated week 3 foods and the *Foods to Limit*. Remember to be especially kind to yourself during this process, taking time to celebrate successes and giving yourself grace when barriers pop up.

WEEK 4: PROTEINS — FISH AND POULTRY

Welcome to week 4! You are halfway there. This week will focus on lean proteins—fish and poultry—in addition to the *Foods to Limit*. It will also offer an opportunity to make mealtimes easier by doing some meal preparation.

What about vegetarians and vegans? It's important to point out here that even moderate adherence to the MIND diet can offer protective benefits to the brain, and those who choose not to eat animal protein can absolutely still follow the MIND diet. Therefore, this week we will offer modifications for you if you follow a vegetarian or vegan diet.

Week 4 Self-Monitoring: Track fish and poultry plus the *Foods to Limit* by using the MIND Diet Refrigerator Chart.

In addition to continuing to track the *Foods to Limit*, here are your targets for this week:

Proteins	MIND Food Points	
Fish & Seafood (Fsh) **Goal:** 1 serving/week **Serving size:** 3–5 ounces	0 servings/week	0
	1+ servings/week	1
Poultry (Poul) **Goal:** 2 servings/week **Serving size:** 3–5 ounces without skin/bones	0 servings/week	0
	1 serving/week	0.5
	2+ servings/week	1

If you follow a vegetarian diet and you're feeling ambitious, you could get a head start on next week's goal to track whole grains and beans. Alternatively, you could choose a group that you may need to improve from weeks 1 through 3. As for tracking other foods, this, again, is up to you. The more you track and plan ahead, the easier it will be to establish habits for the long term—well beyond the 6-week program.

Week 4 Meal Planning: Now is the time to schedule your menu items for the week for fish and poultry servings. This week, we encourage you to continue to plan for dinners as well as routine, consistent breakfasts and lunches. If you feel like you are in a groove with tracking and meal planning, go ahead and schedule the other MIND foods covered in weeks 2 and 3 into your menu, too. That may be more realistic this week since you just need 3 meals or snacks to get to your target for this week's MIND foods! Pick a few recipes to add to your menu, make your grocery list, and go shopping on your scheduled day. Has this become a habit yet or might a new reminder on your calendar be helpful? Take this time to really refine what works for you in terms of finding recipes and scheduling menus. If you find that planning ahead is working well, you may also want to begin using the time you've scheduled for meal prep to make mealtimes more efficient. This could include preparing marinades for these proteins, making dressings for sides, or washing, chopping, and portioning vegetables that might be used as ingredients for salads or sides to accompany the main-course fish and poultry for this week.

Week 4 Action Planning:

WEEK 4 ACTION PLAN

Small Goal #1: Track fish and poultry, plus the *Foods to Limit*. Tally your MIND points at the end of the week and check with the MIND target for each tracked food.

Small Goal #2: Schedule fish and poultry into your menu. Consider recipes that could help build your weekly menu. Make a grocery list and go shopping on your scheduled day to be prepared to incorporate these foods into your routine. Meal prep for your menu items up to 3 days ahead.

If you do need to eliminate fish and/or poultry due to an allergy or special diet restriction, you can modify the goals this week to include other sources of protein in your menu. For example, you can incorporate soybeans or tofu, or combine foods that together form complete proteins, such as pairing whole-grain rice with beans, or barley with lentils. You might also consider talking to your doctor about adding an omega-3 fish oil or plant-based supplement such as flaxseed or walnut oil to get in your DHA/ALA; however, remember that there is not strong evidence to date that plant-based supplementation or use of any supplements is effective in reducing the risk of cognitive decline. Always speak with your doctor before beginning a new supplement to ensure that it does not interact with any other medications or supplements you may be taking, and to make sure it is a good fit for your lifestyle overall.

What about plant-based meat alternatives? The plant-based meat industry is having a big moment. Some brands, such as Beyond Meat and Impossible Foods, offer meat alternatives that are highly processed and high in saturated fat and sodium. So, even though they are labeled "vegan and plant-based," they are not necessarily better for you than regular red meat (though they may be better for the environment). If you choose to consume these meat alternatives, consume them in moderation. If you're looking for plant-based sources of protein, we recommend choosing foods that have gone through the least amount of processing, such as whole grains, nuts, beans, legumes, and tofu. There are many high-protein plant-based foods that are made with minimal processing and can be good alternatives to meat, such as tofu, tempeh, and seitan. In fact, these are staples in many countries where people do not consume a lot of meat.

Week 4 Reflection: In week 4, you will reflect on how your surroundings may be influencing your eating patterns. Research shows that food choices and eating behaviors can be influenced by environmental, social, and psychological factors.[1] Let's break these down.

How does your environment impact your food choices? If you are often surrounded by unhealthy foods such as sweet treats, sugar-sweetened beverages, and fried foods, or tend to dine out more often than preparing meals from home, you'll be more likely to choose these unhealthy options over healthier ones. It could be valuable not only to take inventory of the foods in your home, but to reflect on what foods are available to you throughout your day. Do you find yourself eating from a coworker's candy jar several times per day, sipping on sodas or sweetened coffee drinks, or ordering from fast food menus? The good news is that research shows people who have more fruits and vegetables in the home and those who take time to read food labels tend to have healthier diets. The recommendation is to focus on finding ways to increase healthier options, rather than getting in a restrictive mindset to eliminate all the not-so-healthy ones. If you notice that you're often missing the *Foods to Limit* targets, we suggest revisiting some of the key *Foods to Choose* to ensure those targets are met, such as leafy greens, other veggies, and berries.

How do the people around you influence your eating habits? As mentioned previously, both healthy and unhealthy habits cluster in social networks. You want your family and friends to be on board with your efforts to build a healthy lifestyle. The people you live with will have an especially big influence on the foods you choose to eat. It can be challenging if not everyone is on board. It is important to verbalize to your loved ones clearly what you need in terms of support. This could mean making a request for keeping fewer cookies and sweets in the house, preparing more home-cooked meals, or getting help with meal planning. Let them know how important this is to you.

Social groups and work environments are influential, too. If you have friends who encourage unhealthy habits or if your workplace isn't the pinnacle of health, you do not need to find new friends or get a new job! Instead, try to steer the socializing to activities that will be mutually beneficial. Ask your friends to go for a hike or a walk through town and grab a protein smoothie. At work, suggest salads and sandwiches for lunch meetings instead of pizza. The more open you are to asking for support when faced with barriers versus believing that challenging situations are beyond your control, the more likely you'll be to build a mutual trust. And you may even find that other people want to support you.

How do you think you're doing in the program so far? The mid-point of the program is a good time to check in with your self-confidence and inner trust. We know that those with a higher level of self-confidence and trust in their ability to achieve their goals are more likely to engage in healthy behaviors. If you're not feeling confident about your progress in this journey so far, you may want to check in to see if you're giving yourself enough credit for your successes. As you reflect, be sure to pat yourself on the back for any progress made, even if you're simply becoming more aware of your habits through paying attention to the different MIND foods each week. If you notice that it is challenging for you to plan out weekly menus or go grocery shopping, it likely means that these activities are not yet habits. This is normal! Remember to reward yourself for your efforts, with honesty and nonjudgment.

How has your support system been working out? This week, reflect on the role of your support system (see key elements in the next section). If it is feeling like a good fit, that is wonderful news. Let your support partner know how helpful they are to you, and share your gratitude. If your partner isn't supportive enough, you may need to have a difficult conversation to change the arrangement or find a new support system. If this is the case, before acting, it may be useful to engage in a gratitude practice. You might begin by reflecting on all the ways your partner or group has been helpful to you, even if it's showing you what you *don't* need.

Week 4 Trust and Support: Now that you're halfway through the program, think about whether your support partner or group is giving you the kind of support you need to experience positive growth. This is especially important if you are feeling frustrated with the program or have expectations for certain results such as weight loss that have not been realized yet.

Here are some key elements you want to see in your support system:

- You engage in healthy behaviors with your partner that encourage your goals, rather than engaging in unhealthy behaviors such as eating out frequently or skipping other planned goals.

- You have conversations that help problem-solve the obstacles and barriers that you are having as opposed to conversations that rationalize unhealthy behaviors or make excuses.

- You receive support without judgment so you can be vulnerable and honest.

- Your partner shows up consistently for meetups or scheduled phone calls.

- Your partner engages in plenty of conversation with you that helps you grow and achieve your goals. They listen well and understand what is needed to help you move forward. If there is lingering confusion or unanswered questions, it may be a sign that the type of support is insufficient. If your support partner is a peer — that is, someone on a similar journey — you may need more of a professional coach to guide you.

WEEK 4 WEIGHT LOSS ON THE MIND

BONUS TOOLS FOR WEIGHT LOSS:

Nutrition Tracking App

Body Weight Scale

Meal Timing Schedule

Lifestyle Program or Health Coach

Reflect on past refrigerator charts or feedback from a nutrition tracking app to provide clues on how to maximize weight loss.

Consider a meal timing schedule. People who eat breakfast daily, plan ahead for balanced meals, and avoid late-night eating are more likely to lose weight.

Incorporate regular physical activity.

Consider added support from a lifestyle program or health coach.

Now is a good time to note any progress in your weight loss. Remember that a healthy rate of weight loss is anywhere from ½ pound to 2 pounds per week. If you're seeing progress, congrats! Try not to get discouraged if you're not seeing consistent loss. Instead, here are a few suggestions for exploring how you can enhance your weight loss efforts:

- **Take inventory of tracked foods.** I recommend looking back at your previous food charts. They may help explain why you're not seeing the results you may have expected by now. Remember that the *Foods to Limit* are not only harmful to the brain and heart; they are also much more calorie-dense. If you're using a nutrition tracking app, you may have noticed that these calories add up very quickly. Consider whether you may be going over the recommended targets.

  You might also check in to see how thorough you've been in tracking foods. Remember that research shows that people are more successful with weight loss when they keep complete food records. So, if your trackers look sparse, you might try to be more MINDful about recording your intake in the upcoming weeks.

- **Consider a meal timing schedule.** As previously mentioned, the following factors were shown to play a significant role in weight loss:

  - *Breakfast*: Breakfast eaters are more likely to be at a healthy weight, and people who have successfully lost and maintained weight report that they eat breakfast daily.

  - *Balanced meals plus snacks*: Some research suggests that three balanced meals and one or two snacks a day is ideal. We recommend starting with breakfast within 2 hours of waking and then paying attention to your hunger cues.

o *Avoiding late-night eating:* Late-night eating is thought to be particularly harmful for sleep patterns, weight loss efforts, and overall health and well-being.

o *Intermittent fasting:* We don't recommend this method every day, but trying it for 2 or 3 days per week may help you with your weight loss efforts. Review chapter 16 for a refresher on intermittent fasting and other tips for meal timing.

o *Repetition of foods or meals:* Repeating meals and snacks throughout the week can be an easy way to plan, and some research shows that reducing the variability of meals may help with weight loss efforts. You could do this by rotating two or three breakfast ideas for the week, planning to make just two dinner recipes and eating leftovers for another two lunches and dinners, or keeping the same two or three snack ideas in rotation for the week.

- **Schedule regular physical activity.** Physical activity is a crucial ingredient to weight loss, especially for sustained weight loss. Consider whether you are moving enough each day and remember that this can be as simple as adding moderate-intensity walking to your regular routine. Revisit chapter 17 for ways to customize an exercise routine that is right for you.

- **Consider expert support.** If you're considering upgrading to a more professional level of support, we recommend finding a lifestyle program offered through your fitness club or community center, or working with a professional health coach such as a registered dietitian nutritionist. This does not necessarily mean that you abandon your previous support partner. It's okay to have an additional layer of support. Professional support can be especially useful in helping you achieve your weight loss goal by guiding you through barriers and strategies you may not have been able to identify on your own. Turn to chapter 16 for tips on connecting to additional support. Don't be afraid to ask for help—a little extra support can go a long way!

WEEK 5: CARBOHYDRATES — WHOLE GRAINS AND BEANS

Welcome to week 5! This is the time to push past any fatigue and focus on your small steps to really commit to health. This week, we tackle the healthy carbohydrates—whole grains and beans. You can use the MIND Plate for Meal Planning to ensure your menu options are balanced. We also add tracking of wine as an option to incorporate, with the reminder that you should not increase alcohol consumption if you are not currently a drinker.

Week 5 Self-Monitoring: Track whole grains, beans, wine, and the *Foods to Limit* using the MIND Diet Refrigerator Chart.

In addition to continuing to track the *Foods to Limit*, here are your targets for this week:

Carbohydrates	MIND Food Points	
Whole Grains (WG) **Goal:** 3 servings/day **Serving size:** 1 slice bread or ½ cup cooked grains	0–4 servings/week	0
	5–20 servings/week	0.5
	21+ servings/week	1
Beans & Legumes (Bn) **Goal:** 3 servings/week **Serving size:** ½ cup canned or cooked	0 servings/week	0
	1–2 servings/week	0.5
	3+ servings/week	1

Moderation	MIND Food Points	
Wine (Win) **Goal:** 1 serving/day **Serving size:** 5 fluid ounces	0 servings/week	0
	1–6 servings/week	0.5
	7 servings/week	1
	8+ servings/week	0.5

If you've been doing well tracking all the MIND foods we've covered so far, you should keep this up! Otherwise, you can keep focus on just the designated MIND foods for this week.

Week 5 Meal Planning: Now is the time to plan your intake of whole grains and beans. Just as we encouraged last week, you can continue menu planning for dinners, breakfasts, and lunches if you're getting into the swing of that. When you write out your weekly menu, schedule in meals that incorporate the MIND foods for the week and, if you are in a rhythm, plan menu items incorporating the other MIND diet foods, too; the more you practice this, the easier it will become. The target for whole grains is 3 servings per day; if you don't eat them regularly, start with 1 or 2 servings per day of a whole grain you like. Remember, a serving of whole grains is only 1 slice whole-grain bread or ½ cup cooked grains, so it might be easier than you think to get your servings in.

You can also choose some recipes to add to your menu, make your grocery list, get your shopping done, and then determine what menu items could benefit from meal prep. Continue to evaluate whether these activities have become habits or if you need other support, such as reminders in your calendar. You may want to incorporate the MIND Plate for Meal Planning this week. By now, you'll likely have ideas for how to incorporate the foods that make up a complete MIND Plate, since the healthy carbohydrate group is the last component to bring balance to a meal when combined with the foods from weeks 2 through 4 (½ plate vegetables/fruit + 2 thumbs healthy fats + ¼ plate lean protein + ¼ plate healthy carbs). Review chapter 15 for a full recap and menu-planning ideas with the MIND Plate.

If this feels overwhelming and you're still establishing good habits of self-monitoring and scheduling menu items with the MIND foods of the week, then you can just focus on planning a few meals with the intention of incorporating healthy carbs and continue to use your refrigerator chart to mark just your whole grains and beans/legumes plus the *Foods to Limit* this week.

Week 5 Action Planning:

WEEK 5 ACTION PLAN

Small Goal #1: Track whole grains, beans/legumes, wine, and the *Foods to Limit*. Tally your MIND points at the end of the week and check it with the MIND target for each tracked food.

Small Goal #2: Schedule whole grains and beans/legumes into your menu. Consider recipes that could help build your weekly menu. Make a grocery list and go shopping on your scheduled day to be prepared to incorporate these foods into your routine. Meal prep for menu items up to 3 days ahead. Also consider using the MIND Plate for Meal Planning to balance meals.

Week 5 Reflection: This week, **focus on how you feel after consuming the moderation foods compared to when you have meals that are mostly plant-based and well balanced.** The moderation foods include wine and the *Foods to Limit*. Notice whether you tend to overindulge in these foods, especially wine. Pay attention to thoughts, emotions, and physical sensations after consuming the moderation foods. Do you experience any mood changes, digestive issues, or changes in your energy levels immediately or even up to 12 hours after? It's important to connect what you eat to how you feel. Try to do this without judgment or shame; those feelings will not help you progress.

You should also review, modify, and recommit to your small goals this week by reflecting on all of your past small goals since week 1. Take a moment to reflect on what is going well and what might feel challenging. Instead of focusing too much on the outcome, be kind to yourself and identify ways to stay motivated. Don't forget that the last step in the reflection process is to generate your gratitude list of five new things you're feeling thankful for; this can help you put things into perspective and maintain your momentum.

Week 5 Trust and Support: This week, consider how you might be able to harness the power of your support network to strengthen your new habits. If you have a number of people in your household, ask them to help with some of the planning, shopping, and meal prep. This can be especially fun for kids if they choose part of the meal; it can also model great nutrition habits early on. If you live alone, you might create a balanced MIND meal and invite your support partner over for lunch or dinner. If you're on this journey with a group of peers, it could be fun and motivating to have everyone bring a balanced MIND dish to a potluck-style meal.

You could also simply share your successes with your partner and, if you're having trouble with anything, ask them to check in on you later in the week. For example, if you've been doing well tracking your MIND foods and shopping for groceries but are falling short on preparing balanced meals, a check-in at or around a mealtime could help identify how the breakdown happens.

WEEK 5 WEIGHT LOSS ON THE MIND

BONUS TOOLS FOR WEIGHT LOSS:

Nutrition Tracking App

Body Weight Scale

Meal Timing Schedule

Lifestyle Program or Health Coach

Self-reflect on the connection between the moderation foods, including wine and the *Foods to Limit,* and your weight patterns.

Consider tracking *all* alcohol consumed and aim for 1 or fewer drinks per day. Excess intake of alcohol of any kind may prevent you from losing weight.

As you check in on your weight this week, see if you can connect any discoveries in your self-reflection with your weight patterns. You may have already discovered a connection between the more calorie-dense foods on the *Foods to Limit* list and your weight. Also consider wine and other alcohol consumed, even if you're not recording all alcoholic beverages. Drinking excess alcohol of any kind is likely to limit your ability to lose weight for several reasons. First, it's high in calories and provides few nutrients. You might also notice that you're likely to eat more, and eat more unhealthy foods, when you're drinking, since alcohol lowers your inhibitions and can impact your judgment.

If you do discover a connection between the moderation foods and your weight, such as not making weight loss progress on the weeks you exceed the wine or sweets targets, consider scaling back to track just those items for the next week, or devote a week to making substitutions for those habits to test whether they could impact your weight. You might try swapping out your evening wine or dessert a few nights per week for herbal tea or an alcohol-free spritzer made of sparkling water, berries, and a twist of lemon or lime. Be kind to yourself and feel confident that these things don't have to change overnight.

WEEK 6: PROGRAM REFLECTION AND YOUR ROADMAP TO MINDFUL LIVING

Congratulations, you made it to the final week! This week is all about examining what went well and what could be improved so that you can choose which healthy habits to carry forward to create your own roadmap for a MINDful life.

As we've said many times but can't emphasize enough: creating an individualized approach to the habits we have covered in this program is key to your success in sustaining an optimal lifestyle for cognitive health and longevity. To help with this, we offer 2 weeks of sample meal plans in the appendix (page 337) and encourage you to customize these according to what you've learned over the past 6 weeks. This could mean swapping some of the MIND foods to fit your food preferences or cultural practices or changing the number of times you eat per day.

Week 6 Self-Monitoring: Now is the time to reflect on the last 5 weeks by reviewing your food charts from the previous weeks. The foods that need the most improvement will be your focus this week. If you scored 0 to 0.5 points in any of the categories, note these foods as areas for possible attention. Ending the program as it began, track all the MIND diet foods once again, this time with an eye toward making improvements to your overall eating pattern. Comparing this week's MIND diet score to week 1 will tell you if you've improved your predicted risk for Alzheimer's disease over the past 6 weeks.

Week 6 Meal Planning: By this week you probably have a good idea of what days and times work for the meal-planning activities of scheduling your weekly menu, making a grocery list and shopping, and meal preparation. If you feel this process isn't refined yet, that's okay! Life is fluid and your routines will need to adjust to whatever life is throwing your way. You can customize your own roadmap, as the habit of meal planning will look different for everyone.

Aim to menu plan with the *Foods to Choose* that need improvement and try to find substitutes for the *Foods to Limit* so you can stay within a brain- and heart-healthy range of consumption. For example, if your red meat intake is high, substitute a couple of meals with chicken or beans, or swap in EVOO for cooking or avocado as a spread in place of butter. If you consistently ate more than one fried food meal each week, experiment with sushi or healthier fast food like freshly made salads and sandwiches from a local shop. The more nourishing substitutes you find, the easier it will become! For those recipes you've chosen and foods you've scheduled in your menu, make your grocery list and determine your shopping day, along with the menu items you will meal prep up to 3 days ahead.

Week 6 Action Planning:

WEEK 6 ACTION PLAN

Small Goal #1: Track all MIND diet foods: Use your MIND Diet Refrigerator Charts from weeks 1–5 to identify the food(s) that need improvement. Tally your MIND points at the end of the week for each food and compare your week 6 MIND diet score to your week 1 MIND diet score. Record in your journal.

Small Goal #2: Schedule the *Foods to Choose* that need improvement into your menu and find healthy substitutes for the *Foods to Limit* as needed. Consider recipes that could help build your weekly menu. Make a grocery list and go shopping on your scheduled day to be prepared to incorporate these foods into your routine. Meal prep for your menu items up to 3 days ahead. Also consider using the MIND Plate for Meal Planning to balance meals.

Week 6 Reflection: In week 6, **examine the practices that help you stay on track, motivate you, and keep you energized.** Begin by reviewing all of your past journal reflection entries from weeks 1–5. Does eating a veggie-loaded breakfast in the morning help you make better food choices throughout the day? Do you find that having an afternoon green protein smoothie and a brisk walk increases energy better than a sweet treat? Really lean into these practices and try to make them more habitual.

If overindulging in the *Foods to Limit* is an issue, take time to home in on the factors and events that lead to this behavior. Examine the environment in which you consume these foods, the hunger cues surrounding them, the eating triggers, and the physical feelings you get from eating them. Acknowledge what could use improvement and identify solutions that you could try.

Week 6 Trust and Support: Since this is the last week and we want to finish strong, we will focus on why it was hard to reach the target and what steps are needed to improve. Your support partner or group could be a particularly good resource this week in helping you think this through. This week, when meeting with your support network, be sure to fully express any challenges you have encountered and ask for help where it is needed. Start looking beyond your support partner and expand to the people around you. Sometimes the little act of saying it out loud can help you find solutions.

WEEK 6 WEIGHT LOSS ON THE MIND

BONUS TOOLS FOR WEIGHT LOSS:

Nutrition Tracking App

Body Weight Scale

Meal Timing Schedule

Lifestyle Program or Health Coach

Sugar-sweetened beverages can block your ability to lose weight, as they can be a significant source of empty calories.

A weight loss goal of 5–10% could take up to 6–12 months. Repeat the 6-week program as many times as needed to establish healthy habits and achieve your long-term weight loss goal.

If you've been tracking all the MIND foods or focused on the moderation foods last week and found that you consistently drank more wine than one glass daily or indulged in more than four sweets servings, it may be time to create some new habits. The same is true if you noticed an excess of sugar-sweetened beverages, especially if you're interested in weight loss. These types of sweet drinks have been linked not only to obesity but also to adverse health conditions such as heart disease and diabetes. Remember to track all beverages that contribute calories, including juices, smoothies and shakes, and specialty coffee drinks and teas. The good news is that it can be easy to mimic these types of drinks without all the added sugar. You might consider a replacement such as sparkling water, herbal tea, or even MIND-friendly plain water with fresh or frozen berries.

If you've been monitoring your intake via a nutrition tracking app, you will find a variety of nutritional reports and trend summaries that can help you determine your areas for improvement.

When checking in with your weight this week, it's good to take a look at the trend from week 1 until now, but keep in mind that it may not be realistic for you to reach your goal without continued efforts. We recommend reflecting on what worked best for you over the course of the 6 weeks and setting the intention to continue the most helpful behaviors going forward. When striving for sustained weight loss, a 12-week period of consistently practicing new habits is often needed. Remember that an initial weight loss goal of 5 to 10 percent could take 6 to 12 months.

The Official MIND Diet 6-Week Program is designed to give you the tools you need to establish habits around healthy eating for a MINDful life. The beauty of the MIND diet is that anyone can incorporate it into their existing lifestyle. You could continue following it for as long as it takes for the new habits to become automatic. Or, you might decide to go back and focus only on certain weeks. For example, maybe you are not getting in your EVOO, and you decide to go back to week 3 to do it again.

You can also revisit the program anytime you feel like your eating has slipped or you need a boost of motivation. We recommend beginning with the MIND Diet Quiz and focusing on either simply tracking your intake using the refrigerator chart or repeating the 6-week program. Find a buddy to do the program with you or host a cookbook club highlighting recipes for each of the MIND diet foods.

Most of all, remember that the way you eat is very personal, and changing it takes time and intention. Approaching this process without judgment is the best way forward to healthy living. Be proud of and reward yourself when you make choices that align with your intention to live a healthy life. It's important to remember that diet alone does not equal health. In addition to a healthy diet, engaging in regular physical activity, getting good-quality sleep, fostering positive social interactions, learning new things, and having a positive outlook on life are practices we should all strive for to have optimal health and longevity.

> "No single food will make or break good health. But the kinds of food you choose day in and day out will have major impact."
>
> —*Walter Willett*

PART V

THE MIND DIET RECIPES

By Laura Morris

"Food, family, and the camaraderie of meals is central to the expression of love."

—Dr. Martha Clare Morris

CHAPTER 19

Your Kitchen, Your Home

When I was a kid, we had a routine that happened every week of every month of every year. On Saturday mornings my parents would sit down and write out a weekly dinner menu, then make out a grocery list of all the foods we would need. My dad was usually tasked with making the trip to the store, and he'd often take me along. This time was so special. I got to be with my dad, one on one, doing something we both loved to do, which was serving our family through food. Both my parents worked full-time jobs, and eating well was a top priority. So this ritual of preparing for the week's meals was important.

My father typically got home first from work, so he was the top chef in our house. He would chop, sauté, steam, and bake nutritious meals every weekday (my mother often cooked on the weekends). No matter what day of the week it was, the menu revolved around whole grains, vegetables, beans, and seafood, and of course lots of extra-virgin olive oil. Helping my dad in the kitchen had a huge influence on me, as it led me to my career as a nutrition consultant and chef.

I am often asked how I got into cooking. Like many people in the culinary world, I love food. I also love nutrition, as it was foundational to my upbringing. When I was working in clinical nutrition, educating people on what foods to eat and why, I felt that there must be something more I could offer people beyond just teaching them

237

about protein, carbohydrates, fats, vitamins, and minerals. Now, don't get me wrong, this knowledge is vital. But it is just one piece of the pie. Food is a universal language we all speak. Not only is eating central to many of our holidays and celebrations, it's also something we do multiple times on an ordinary day. It is undoubtedly one of our greatest pleasures in life and should be a highlight of each day, not just something you check off your to-do list. I've always known this instinctively, of course, but something happened in my early adulthood that really showed me the crucial role that food plays in our lives.

When I was 25 years old, my father was diagnosed with stage 4 esophageal cancer. Very early in his 4-year battle, he lost his ability to eat by mouth and was reliant on a feeding tube to get all his nutrition. Our house chef, lover of food, and creator of meals could no longer participate in one of our most cherished rituals—gathering around the table for a delicious meal. I became consumed with figuring out how he could regain his ability to eat. At that point, I was determined to connect with food on a deeper level, so I enrolled in culinary school and began a journey that would shape my life.

At first, Dad was too weak and ill to take care of our family's food needs, so I willingly stepped in to cook dinners and holiday meals and host parties. Yet a surprising thing happened. My father loved hanging out in the kitchen and being in on the action, so on days he had the strength, he stepped in and cooked along with me. I taught him what I had been learning in school, and together we would create beautiful dinners. Although he couldn't eat, my father found a way to participate in the process, which was so special to him and our whole family.

Although he never did regain his ability to eat, he would occasionally take little tastes here and there of our creations. Working in the kitchen with my dad—talking, laughing, connecting over something we both loved—gave me happy memories that I will cherish forever. Cooking also took my sadness and worry over his illness and gave it purpose in my life.

I believe food and cooking are so much greater than just nutrition;

they're a way to connect with your loved ones. It's in that spirit that I share these recipes with you. Many are versions of dishes I grew up eating; some are variations of recipes I cooked with my dad. They are curated with not only a deep understanding of nutrition but also a real passion for food and its ability to nourish you and your loved ones. I hope you find a way to use these recipes and adjust them to your tastes and family traditions.

Each recipe in the following five chapters shows you the MIND diet points per serving, using this legend:

LG: leafy green vegetables
OV: other vegetables
Ber: berries
EVOO: extra-virgin olive oil
Nut: nuts and seeds
Fsh: fish and seafood
Poul: poultry
WG: whole grains
Bn: beans and legumes

CHAPTER 20

Breakfast

Veggie Frittata

MIND POINTS: 1 SERVING = 1 LG, 1 OV, 0.5 EVOO

Frittatas are one of the best ways to use up veggies in your refrigerator. You can use any veggies, such as zucchini, bell peppers, eggplant, kale, spinach, Swiss chard, etc. This meal is great when hosting a brunch or for a light, delicious dinner. I love to top a frittata with raw leafy greens for added texture and freshness.

Serves: 8
Prep time: 10 minutes
Cook time: 30 minutes

12 large eggs

4 tablespoons extra-virgin olive oil

1 medium sweet potato, peeled and cut into small dice

1 teaspoon Old Bay Seasoning

1 medium red onion, thinly sliced

4 cups chopped Tuscan kale

4 garlic cloves, thinly sliced

¼ teaspoon salt

¼ teaspoon black pepper

Preheat the oven to 400°F.

In a large bowl, gently whisk the eggs until just incorporated; set aside.

In a large cast-iron skillet or other oven-safe skillet, heat 2 tablespoons of the oil over medium heat. Add the sweet potato and Old Bay and cook, stirring frequently, until crispy and cooked through, about 7 minutes. Transfer the sweet potato to a plate.

Add the remaining 2 tablespoons oil to the pan. When hot, add the onion and cook, stirring frequently, until translucent and slightly browned, about 4 minutes. Add the kale, garlic, salt, and pepper and cook, stirring, for 2 to 3 minutes, until the kale begins to wilt.

Return the sweet potato to the pan. Add the eggs and stir lightly. Turn the heat down to low and cook, without stirring, for 5 to 7 minutes, until the eggs begin to set.

Transfer the pan to the oven and bake for 10 minutes, or until the eggs are cooked through in the center. Cut into 8 wedges to serve.

Nutritional analysis per serving (serving size: 1 slice): Calories: 230, Total Fat: 14 g, Saturated Fat: 3 g, Trans fat: 0 g, Polyunsaturated Fat: 2 g, Monounsaturated Fat: 8 g, Cholesterol: 250 mg, Sodium: 370 mg, Total Carbohydrates: 16 g, Dietary Fiber: 3 g, Total Sugars: 3 g (including 0 g added sugar), Protein: 11 g

Veggie Hash with Eggs

MIND POINTS: 1 SERVING = 2 OV, 1 EVOO, 1 WG

A good breakfast hash is such a great way to get a hearty meal in while using whatever veggies you have on hand. Just sauté up the veggies, add a leftover grain, and top with eggs—it's that simple! This recipe uses quinoa, but any grain will work.

Serves: 2
Prep time: 10 minutes
Cook time: 20 minutes

3 tablespoons extra-virgin olive oil

1 medium sweet potato, peeled and cut into ½-inch dice

⅓ cup sliced red onion

2 cups roughly chopped broccoli florets

¼ teaspoon salt

¼ teaspoon black pepper

1 cup cooked quinoa

2 large eggs

2 tablespoons chopped fresh chives (optional)

2 tablespoons salsa (optional)

1 teaspoon hot sauce (optional)

Heat 2 tablespoons of the oil in a large skillet over medium heat. Add the sweet potato and cook, stirring occasionally, for 5 to 7 minutes, until slightly browned but still firm on the inside.

Add the onion, broccoli, salt, and pepper and cook for 5 minutes, or until the broccoli is fork-tender and the sweet potato is cooked through. Add the quinoa and stir to warm through, about 2 minutes. Transfer the mixture to a serving bowl.

Add the remaining 1 tablespoon oil to the pan. When hot, crack the eggs into the pan one at a time. Turn the heat down to low and cook the eggs until the whites are mostly set and the yolk begins to slightly thicken, about 2 minutes. Flip each egg and cook until just set, another 10 to 30 seconds. Transfer the eggs to the top of the vegetable hash. Serve warm, topped with your favorite garnishes.

Nutritional analysis per serving (serving size: 1 egg + ½ hash): Calories: 380, Total Fat: 20 g, Saturated Fat: 3 g, Trans fat: 0 g, Polyunsaturated Fat: 3 g, Monounsaturated Fat: 12 g, Cholesterol: 165 mg, Sodium: 400 mg, Total Carbohydrates: 39 g, Dietary Fiber: 5 g, Total Sugars: 6 g (including 0 g added sugar), Protein: 13 g

Olive Oil Veggie Scramble

MIND POINTS: 1 SERVING = 0.5 LG, 1 OV, 1 EVOO

A veggie scramble is an easy, no-fuss meal anytime of the day. It is also a great way to get in a couple servings of veggies. Think of this as a "use what you have in the fridge" recipe—almost no veggie is off limits; just be sure to cut them into small, uniform pieces. Enjoy as is or with whole-grain toast and a side of berries.

Serves: 2
Prep time: 10 minutes
Cook time: 5 minutes

2 tablespoons extra-virgin olive oil

¼ cup diced yellow onion

½ cup diced orange bell pepper

½ cup diced tomato

1 garlic clove, chopped

1 cup spinach leaves, cut into chiffonade

4 large eggs, beaten

Pinch salt (optional)

Pinch black pepper (optional)

In a medium skillet, heat the oil over medium heat. Add the onion, bell pepper, and tomato and sauté until tender, 2 to 3 minutes. Add the garlic and sauté until fragrant, 1 to 2 minutes. Add the spinach and cook just until wilted, about 1 minute.

Add the eggs and cook, using a silicone spatula to scrape the set eggs from the bottom of the pan and allow the loose eggs to cook. Continue scrambling until the eggs are mostly set, about 1 minute. Turn off the heat and stir the eggs for another minute, until they are cooked to the desired doneness. Season with salt and pepper, if desired.

Nutritional analysis per serving (serving size: 1 cup): Calories: 260, Total Fat: 21 g, Saturated Fat: 4 g, Trans fat: 0 g, Polyunsaturated Fat: 3 g, Monounsaturated Fat: 13 g, Cholesterol: 280 mg, Sodium: 280 mg, Total Carbohydrates: 7 g, Dietary Fiber: 2 g, Total Sugars: 2 g (including 0 g added sugar), Protein: 11 g

Loaded Breakfast Sandwich

MIND POINTS: 1 SERVING = 0.5 LG, 1 OV, 1 WG

A breakfast sandwich is always a favorite for a hungry morning. You can use any veggies you have on hand, such as cooked zucchini, bell peppers, or onions; just be sure to cut them into thin slices. This recipe uses pesto as a tasty spread, but you could substitute smashed avocado, hummus, or a light cheese such as Swiss.

Serves: 2
Prep time: 5 minutes
Cook time: 10 minutes

> 1 tablespoon extra-virgin olive oil
>
> 1 cup sliced mushrooms
>
> 1 tablespoon balsamic vinegar
>
> ¼ teaspoon salt
>
> 2 large eggs
>
> 2 tablespoons Arugula Pesto (page 314)
>
> 2 whole-wheat English muffins, toasted
>
> 4 tomato slices

Heat ½ tablespoon of the oil in a large skillet over medium heat. Add the mushrooms and sauté for 4 minutes, stirring occasionally to get a nice brown color. Add the balsamic vinegar and salt, stir, and continue to cook for another 2 to 3 minutes. Transfer the mushrooms to a plate.

Add the remaining ½ tablespoon oil to the pan. When hot, crack the eggs in, one at a time. Turn the heat down to low and cook the eggs until the whites are mostly set, about 2 minutes. Flip the eggs and cook for another minute, or until they reach the desired doneness. Turn off the heat.

Spread ½ tablespoon pesto onto each English muffin half. Top 2 muffin halves with an egg. Divide the mushrooms and tomato slices on top of the eggs, and close with the other muffin half.

Nutritional analysis per serving (serving size: 1 sandwich): Calories: 370, Total Fat: 22 g, Saturated Fat: 4 g, Trans fat: 0 g, Polyunsaturated Fat: 4 g, Monounsaturated Fat: 12 g, Cholesterol: 190 mg, Sodium: 750 mg, Total Carbohydrates: 30 g, Dietary Fiber: 5 g, Total Sugars: 8 g (including 1 g added sugar), Protein: 14 g

Bonus Peanut Butter Toast

MIND POINTS: 1 SERVING = 1 BER, 0.5 NUT, 1 WG

Peanut butter toast is my go-to breakfast and was for my mother as well. It is so easy and provides healthy fats, protein, and carbohydrates to start your day. I love to add brain-healthy berries and hemp seeds to make it "bonus" toast. Pear or apple slices also work well, with a pinch of ground cinnamon.

Serves: 2
Prep time: 5 minutes

2 tablespoons natural peanut butter

2 slices whole-grain bread, toasted

1 cup berries of choice, sliced

1 tablespoon hemp seeds

Spread 1 tablespoon peanut butter on each slice of toast and top with ½ cup berries and ½ tablespoon hemp seeds.

Nutritional analysis per serving (serving size: 1 toast): Calories: 250, Total Fat: 12 g, Saturated Fat: 1.5 g, Trans fat: 0 g, Polyunsaturated Fat: 4.5 g, Monounsaturated Fat: 5 g, Cholesterol: 0 mg, Sodium: 180 mg, Total Carbohydrates: 26 g, Dietary Fiber: 3 g, Total Sugars: 9 g (including 0 g added sugar), Protein: 9 g

Fancy Smoked Salmon Toast

MIND POINTS: 1 SERVING = 0.5 LG, 0.5 FSH, 1 WG

I love the smoky, buttery, delicate taste of smoked salmon. This dish adds spicy arugula and tart pickled onions to make you feel like you are eating at a fancy restaurant. If you want to make this dish a little lighter, you can substitute hummus for the avocado as a spread and add sliced cucumbers. I often make this as a quick, delicious lunch. You can find packages of smoked salmon in the seafood section at most grocery stores.

Serves: 2
Prep time: 5 minutes

   1 ripe avocado, halved and pitted

   2 slices whole-grain bread, toasted

   1 cup arugula

   4 ounces smoked salmon

   2 tablespoons Pickled Red Onions (page 320)

   ¼ teaspoon salt

   ¼ teaspoon black pepper

Spread ½ avocado on each piece of toast. Add the arugula to each toast. Layer the smoked salmon on top. Top with the pickled red onions and season with the salt and pepper.

Nutritional analysis per serving (serving size: 1 toast): Calories: 260, Total Fat: 14 g, Saturated Fat: 2 g, Trans fat: 0 g, Polyunsaturated Fat: 2.5 g, Monounsaturated Fat: 8 g, Cholesterol: 15 mg, Sodium: 830 mg, Total Carbohydrates: 19 g, Dietary Fiber: 5 g, Total Sugars: 2 g (including 0 g added sugar), Protein: 16 g

Hippie Oat Bowls

MIND POINTS: 1 SERVING = 1 BER, 1 NUT, 1 WG

I love these hearty bowls packed with all the delicious seeds and nuts you could ask for. Even if you are not an oatmeal fan, you will love these bowls for breakfast or after a good workout. You can switch up the nuts, seeds, and fruit to whatever is in your pantry. This dish is so filling and energizing! You can also make this the night before and stick it in the refrigerator.

Serves: 1
Prep time: 5 minutes

- ½ cup old-fashioned rolled oats
- 2 tablespoons walnuts or nut of choice
- 1 tablespoon sunflower seeds or hemp seeds
- ½ medium banana, sliced
- ½ cup blueberries or berries of choice
- ½ teaspoon ground cinnamon
- ½ tablespoon cacao nibs (optional)
- ¾ cup milk of choice
- 2 tablespoons dried cranberries (optional)
- 1 teaspoon honey (optional)

In a cereal bowl, layer the oats, walnuts, sunflower seeds, banana, berries, cinnamon, and cacao nibs (if using). Pour the milk over the mixture. Top with the dried cranberries and honey, if desired.

Nutritional analysis per serving (serving size: 1 bowl): Calories: 480, Total Fat: 21 g, Saturated Fat: 3.5 g, Trans fat: 0 g, Polyunsaturated Fat: 11 g, Monounsaturated Fat: 2.5 g, Cholesterol: 0 mg, Sodium: 70 mg, Total Carbohydrates: 63 g, Dietary Fiber: 10 g, Total Sugars: 21 g (including 5 g added sugar), Protein: 17 g

Blueberry Pie Overnight Oats

MIND POINTS: 1 SERVING = 1 BER, 1 NUT, 1 WG

We had a love affair with blueberry pie in my home growing up. It was my mother's favorite dessert, and her recipe was the best around. This breakfast dish is inspired by that family favorite. The oats are toasted before soaking to give them a sweeter, nuttier taste. If you want even more flavor, you can toast the chopped walnuts in the pan with the oats. The blueberries are lightly sweetened with a bit of sugar, which helps create the jam-like texture of the blueberry compote. When you simmer the blueberries, there is no need to add water, as the berries will burst open and provide lots of liquid. I find that a 1:1 ratio of milk to oats is best for a hearty oat texture, but if you want it a bit creamier, you can add another ¼ cup milk. This recipe calls for walnuts, but you can use any nut you prefer.

Serves: 4
Prep time: 10 minutes
Cook time: 10 minutes, plus 4 hours to chill

For the blueberry compote:

    5 cups fresh or frozen blueberries

    1 tablespoon honey

1 tablespoon lemon juice

2 teaspoons sugar

½ teaspoon ground cinnamon

For the oats:

1½ cups old-fashioned rolled oats

½ teaspoon ground cinnamon

¼ teaspoon ground allspice

Pinch ground nutmeg

1½ cups milk of choice

1 cup chopped raw walnuts

In a medium saucepan, combine the blueberries, honey, lemon juice, sugar, and cinnamon. Bring to a simmer over medium heat and cook for 5 to 7 minutes, until some blueberries have burst. Remove from the heat and let cool completely.

While the blueberries are cooking, in a large skillet, combine the oats, cinnamon, allspice, and nutmeg. Toast the oats and spices over medium-low heat, stirring continuously, until the oats are slightly golden and the spices are fragrant, 3 to 5 minutes. Remove from the heat and let cool completely.

Once the oats are cool, transfer to a bowl and stir in the milk.

Layer 4 mason jars or other containers with equal amounts of the oats, chopped nuts, and blueberry compote. Cover and refrigerate for at least 4 hours or as long as 5 days.

Nutritional analysis per serving (serving size: 1 jar): Calories: 490, Total Fat: 24 g, Saturated Fat: 3 g, Trans fat: 0 g, Polyunsaturated Fat: 15 g, Monounsaturated Fat: 3 g, Cholesterol: 5 mg, Sodium: 45 mg, Total Carbohydrates: 78 g, Dietary Fiber: 14 g, Total Sugars: 28 g (including 6 g added sugar), Protein: 18 g

Chia Seed Pudding with Berries

MIND POINTS: 1 SERVING = 1 BER, 1.5 NUT

Who doesn't love an easy-to-grab, delicious breakfast in the morning? Chia seed pudding has been having a moment, and for good reason. Chia seeds are loaded with antioxidants, fiber, healthy fats, and minerals. When soaked in liquid, they become almost creamy, with a pudding-like texture. I make large batches of this pudding and keep it in the refrigerator for quick breakfasts and snacks.

Serves: 6
Prep time: 10 minutes, plus 3 hours to chill

- 1 large ripe banana
- 2 cups oat milk or milk of choice
- ½ cup chia seeds
- ¼ cup pure maple syrup
- 2 tablespoons unsweetened cocoa powder
- 2 tablespoons natural peanut butter or almond butter
- 1 teaspoon vanilla extract
- 3 cups berries of choice
- 1½ cups almonds

In a food processor or blender, blend the banana, milk, chia seeds, maple syrup, cocoa powder, peanut butter, and vanilla until smooth. Divide evenly into six 8-ounce mason jars or small bowls. Cover and refrigerate for at least 3 hours, or for as long as 5 days. Top each jar with ½ cup berries and ¼ cup almonds before serving.

Nutritional analysis per serving (serving size: 1 jar): Calories: 480, Total Fat: 29 g, Saturated Fat: 3 g, Trans fat: 0 g, Polyunsaturated Fat: 5 g, Monounsaturated Fat: 13 g, Cholesterol: 0 mg, Sodium: 55 mg, Total Carbohydrates: 46 g, Dietary Fiber: 15 g, Total Sugars: 22 g (including 10 g added sugar), Protein: 11 g

Key Lime Smoothie

My son Nolan helped me create this smoothie. He loves food that is tart with bright flavors. This smoothie is loaded with spinach to get your day started with a good dose of antioxidants. We make it at least once per week, usually when my spinach is starting to wilt and avocados are getting mushy. You can adjust the amount of ice depending on how frosty you like your smoothies.

Serves: 2
Prep time: 5 minutes

- 2 cups spinach leaves (with stems)
- 1 ripe banana
- 1 ripe avocado, peeled and pitted
- 1 cup milk of choice
- Grated zest and juice of 3 key limes or 1 large lime
- 1 scoop (about ⅓ cup) protein powder
- 1 tablespoon pure maple syrup
- ½ to 1 cup ice

Combine all the ingredients in a blender and blend until smooth and creamy. Pour into 2 glasses.

Nutritional analysis per serving (serving size: 1 smoothie): Calories: 310, Total Fat: 12 g, Saturated Fat: 1.5 g, Trans fat: 0 g, Polyunsaturated Fat: 1.5 g, Monounsaturated Fat: 7 g, Cholesterol: 5 mg, Sodium: 125 mg, Total Carbohydrates: 42 g, Dietary Fiber: 9 g, Total Sugars: 19 g (including 6 g added sugar), Protein: 18 g

Spinach and Coffee Protein Smoothie

MIND POINTS: 1 SERVING = 1 LG

Sometimes, you just need something quick in the morning to give you a little dose of nutrients. Combined with your coffee? Even better! It may seem odd to mix coffee and spinach, but you won't even taste the spinach! This is a quick, no-fuss way to get in your daily leafy greens and an energizing start to your morning. You can also add a banana for a little sweetness and more calories.

Serves 1
Prep time: 5 minutes

- 1 cup spinach leaves (with stems)
- 1 cup milk of choice
- 1 scoop (about ⅓ cup) chocolate or vanilla protein powder
- 1 teaspoon ground coffee or espresso
- 1 cup ice

Combine all the ingredients in a blender and blend until smooth.

Nutritional analysis per serving (serving size: 1 smoothie): Calories: 250, Total Fat: 4 g, Saturated Fat: 0 g, Trans fat: 0 g, Polyunsaturated Fat: 1 g, Monounsaturated Fat: 2 g, Cholesterol: <5 mg, Sodium: 330 mg, Total Carbohydrates: 36 g, Dietary Fiber: 2 g, Total Sugars: 22 g (including 0 g added sugar), Protein: 19 g

Strawberry Green Breakfast Smoothie

MIND POINTS: 1 SERVING = 1 LG, 2 BER, 1 NUT

This sweet, filling smoothie is loaded with brain-healthy foods. Created by Leah, one of the lead dietitians on the MIND diet study, this is a favorite for good reason. You can lighten it up by swapping in water for the milk or omitting the banana and adding extra ice. Frozen berries are great in smoothies as they add a nice thick texture to your drink.

Serves: 1
Prep time: 5 minutes

- 1 cup spinach, kale, or other leafy green
- 1 cup fresh or frozen strawberries
- ½ medium banana
- 2 tablespoons natural peanut butter
- ¾ cup unsweetened vanilla almond milk
- 1 cup ice

Combine all the ingredients in a blender and blend until creamy.

Nutritional analysis per serving (serving size: 1 smoothie): Calories: 390, Total Fat: 20 g, Saturated Fat: 3 g, Trans fat: 0 g, Polyunsaturated Fat: 6 g, Monounsaturated Fat: 10 g, Cholesterol: 0 mg, Sodium: 150 mg, Total Carbohydrates: 35 g, Dietary Fiber: 8 g, Total Sugars: 15 g (including 0 g added sugar), Protein: 16 g

CHAPTER 21

Main Meals

Turkish Tabbouleh with Chicken Meatballs

MIND POINTS: 1 SERVING = 1 OV, 1 EVOO, 1 POUL, 1 WG

Tabbouleh is a popular salad in Middle Eastern cuisines. It is made with bulgur, which comes from cracked wheat that is parboiled and then dried before packaging. It is packed full of vitamins, minerals, and fiber and has a delicious nutty taste and texture. This dish uses tomato paste and a spicy paste called harissa that can be found in the spice section of most grocery stores. The tabbouleh pairs nicely with these savory chicken meatballs. Top with Creamy Tahini Sauce (page 316) or Garlicky Yogurt Sauce (page 315) for a delicious, crowd-pleasing meal—served hot, cold, or at room temperature.

Serves: 4
Prep time: 45 minutes, plus 1 hour to marinate
Cook time: 15 minutes

For the tabbouleh:

    1 cup bulgur, rinsed

    1 cup boiling water

    ¼ cup extra-virgin olive oil

    ¼ cup lemon juice

1 tablespoon tomato paste

2 teaspoons harissa

½ teaspoon salt

1 cup finely chopped cherry tomatoes

1 cup finely chopped cucumber

2 tablespoons diced red onion

¼ cup chopped scallions

⅓ cup chopped fresh parsley

2 tablespoons chopped fresh mint

For the meatballs:

1 pound ground chicken

⅓ cup whole-wheat panko bread crumbs

1 large egg, lightly beaten

2 garlic cloves, chopped

2 tablespoons chopped scallions

1 tablespoon chopped fresh mint

2 teaspoons dried oregano

1 teaspoon ground cumin

1 teaspoon ground allspice

½ teaspoon smoked paprika

½ teaspoon salt

Put the bulgur in a large bowl and carefully pour in the boiling water. Stir.

In a small bowl, whisk together the oil, lemon juice, tomato paste, harissa, and salt. Pour the mixture into the bulgur and stir to incorporate. Let the tabbouleh stand at room temperature for 10 to 15 minutes, until the bulgur has absorbed the liquid. Fluff lightly with a fork.

Stir in the tomatoes, cucumber, red onion, scallions, parsley, and mint. Cover and refrigerate for at least 1 hour or up to overnight.

Preheat the oven to 375°F. Line a rimmed baking sheet with parchment paper or grease it lightly with cooking spray or oil.

In a large bowl, combine all the ingredients for the meatballs. Mix until just incorporated. Using lightly greased hands, roll the mixture into golf-ball-size meatballs. Place them about 2 inches apart on the prepared baking sheet.

Bake for 15 minutes, or until lightly golden brown and cooked through. Serve the meatballs over the tabbouleh.

Nutritional analysis per serving (serving size: 1 cup): Calories: 410, Total Fat: 22 g, Saturated Fat: 4 g, Trans fat: 0 g, Polyunsaturated Fat: 4 g, Monounsaturated Fat: 12 g, Cholesterol: 115 mg, Sodium: 580 mg, Total Carbohydrates: 31 g, Dietary Fiber: 5 g, Total Sugars: 3 g (including 0 g added sugar), Protein: 24 g

Grilled Chicken Spiedies

MIND POINTS: 1 SERVING = 0.5 EVOO, 1 POUL

When I think of spiedies, I think of summer. Whenever one of my aunts comes to visit, they almost always bring a batch of marinating spiedies. This dish originated near my father's hometown in upstate New York and was commonly made with pork. These delicious bites of chicken are tender and juicy, and they have just a little tangy bite from all the lemon and garlic. They are traditionally served with Italian bread, but they go great with just about anything. I like to serve them with Garlicky Yogurt Sauce (page 315) and a hearty salad like the Farro and Arugula Salad (page 294).

Serves: 8
Prep time: 15 minutes, plus 3 hours to chill
Cook time: 10 minutes

¼ cup extra-virgin olive oil

¼ cup red wine vinegar

Juice of 1 lemon

4 garlic cloves, minced

1 tablespoon dried parsley

1½ teaspoons dried oregano

½ teaspoon salt

½ teaspoon black pepper

2 pounds boneless, skinless chicken breast, cut into 1-inch pieces

In a large bowl, whisk together the oil, vinegar, lemon juice, garlic, parsley, oregano, salt, and pepper. Add the chicken and stir to coat well. Cover and refrigerate for at least 3 hours, or up to overnight.

Preheat a grill to high heat. Thread the chicken pieces onto 8 metal skewers (or wooden skewers that have soaked in water for 30 minutes) and grill, turning once, for 5 to 7 minutes, until cooked through. (Alternatively, you can cook the chicken in a large skillet over medium-high heat for 3 to 4 minutes per side, until a golden-brown crust forms and the chicken is cooked through.)

Nutritional analysis per serving (serving size: 1 skewer/4 ounces chicken): Calories: 190, Total Fat: 9 g, Saturated Fat: 1 g, Trans fat: 0 g, Polyunsaturated Fat: 0.5 g, Mono-unsaturated Fat: 5 g, Cholesterol: 65 mg, Sodium: 220 mg, Total Carbohydrates: 1 g, Dietary Fiber: 0 g, Total Sugars: 0 g (including 0 g added sugar), Protein: 26 g

Smoked Paprika Chicken with Seared Green Beans

MIND POINTS: 1 SERVING = 1 OV, 1 POUL

This chicken has bold flavors that really brighten the dish. Add seared green beans and you have an elegant, colorful, and light meal that comes together quickly. If you want to add a sauce, try the Creamy Tahini Sauce on page 316. For a more filling dinner, pair with a salad and whatever grain you have on hand.

Serves: 4
Prep time: 10 minutes
Cook time: 30 minutes

1 tablespoon smoked paprika

1½ teaspoons dried oregano

1½ teaspoons garlic powder

1 teaspoon ground allspice

¼ teaspoon salt

4 (4-ounce) boneless, skinless chicken breasts

2½ tablespoons avocado oil

8 ounces green beans, trimmed

Lime juice (optional)

Preheat the oven to 400°F.

In a small bowl, combine the paprika, oregano, garlic powder, allspice, and salt.

Using a paper towel, pat the chicken breasts dry. Evenly rub the paprika mixture all over the chicken.

Heat 2 tablespoons of the oil in a large skillet over medium-high heat. Add the chicken breasts in a single layer and cook for 4 to 6 minutes, until a light golden crust forms on the bottom. Flip and cook for another 2 to 4 minutes to get a light crust on the other side. Transfer to a rimmed baking sheet.

Bake for 15 to 25 minutes, until the chicken is cooked through—a thermometer inserted in the middle should read 165°F.

Heat the remaining ½ tablespoon oil in the same pan over medium-high heat. Working in batches as necessary so you don't crowd the pan, add the beans in a single layer and cook without stirring for 1 minute, or until they are slightly charred and blistered. Shake the pan or gently roll the beans with tongs and cook for another 1 to 2 minutes without stirring to gently char another side. Turn one more time until the beans are bright green and seared nicely. Transfer to a serving platter.

Squeeze lime juice over the beans, if desired. Serve the chicken over the green beans.

Nutritional analysis per serving (serving size: 1 breast + ½ cup green beans): Calories: 240, Total Fat: 12 g, Saturated Fat: 2 g, Trans fat: 0 g, Polyunsaturated Fat: 2 g, Monounsaturated Fat: 7 g, Cholesterol: 85 mg, Sodium: 370 mg, Total Carbohydrates: 7 g, Dietary Fiber: 3 g, Total Sugars: 1 g (including 0 g added sugar), Protein: 27 g

Saturday Stew

MIND POINTS: 1 SERVING = 1 OV, 0.5 POUL, 1 WG

This is an adaptation of a stew my family ate all the time while I was growing up. We often ate it on Saturday night, so I named it Saturday Stew. It was usually a mishmash of ingredients we had left over from the week. It is flavorful and hearty, and pleases almost all picky eaters. You can make this soup vegan by using veggie grounds in place of the turkey.

Serves: 6
Prep time: 15 minutes
Cook time: 30 minutes

2 tablespoons extra-virgin olive oil

1 pound ground turkey or veggie grounds

1 medium yellow onion, diced

2 medium carrots, peeled and diced

2 garlic cloves, chopped

1 tablespoon dried oregano

1½ teaspoons chopped fresh rosemary

¼ teaspoon dried sage

1 tablespoon Dijon mustard

⅓ cup dry white wine

2 (15-ounce) cans fire-roasted diced tomatoes

6 cups low-sodium vegetable or chicken broth

1 cup fresh, frozen, or drained canned corn

1 bay leaf

2 cups whole-grain elbow macaroni

2 cups chopped kale

⅓ cup grated Parmesan cheese or nutritional yeast (optional)

Heat 1 tablespoon of the oil in a large, heavy-bottomed soup pot over medium heat. Add the turkey or veggie grounds and sauté until lightly golden brown, 5 to 8 minutes for turkey or 4 to 6 minutes for veggie grounds. Transfer to a bowl.

Add the remaining 1 tablespoon oil to the pot. When hot, add the onion and carrots and cook, stirring frequently, until the onion is slightly translucent, 3 to 5 minutes. Stir in the garlic, oregano, rosemary, and sage and cook until fragrant, 1 to 2 minutes. Stir in the mustard to coat the veggies. Add the wine and stir to deglaze the pan. Cook until most of the wine has evaporated, 1 to 2 minutes.

Add the tomatoes with their juices, broth, corn, and bay leaf. Stir and bring to a simmer. Add the macaroni and cook for 8 minutes, or until the macaroni is al dente.

Return the turkey or veggie grounds to the pot, along with the kale. Cook for 2 to 3 minutes, until the kale is just wilted. Remove the bay leaf before serving. Garnish with Parmesan cheese or nutritional yeast, if desired.

Nutritional analysis per serving (serving size: 2 cups): Calories: 360, Total Fat: 10 g, Saturated Fat: 2 g, Trans fat: 0 g, Polyunsaturated Fat: 2 g, Monounsaturated Fat: 5 g, Cholesterol: 35 mg, Sodium: 590 mg, Total Carbohydrates: 46 g, Dietary Fiber: 8 g, Total Sugars: 8 g (including 0 g added sugar), Protein: 22 g

Royal MIND Bowls

MIND POINTS: 1 SERVING = 1 LG, 1 OV, 0.5 EVOO, 0.5 BER, 1 POUL, 0.5 WG, 0.5 BN

This salad, created by Jen, is the ultimate way to get in your MIND foods. You can make it your own by substituting your favorite leafy greens, veggies, grains, berries, nuts, beans, and protein of choice. Or you can eat some version of the salad every day by mixing it up — have nuts on some days, beans on others, poultry or fish on others . . . you get the idea!

Serves: 4
Prep time: 10 minutes

4 cups baby kale

1 cup cooked pearl barley

1 cup chickpeas, drained and rinsed

1 cup small broccoli florets

12 ounces grilled chicken, cut into bite-size pieces

1 cup canned sliced beets

1½ cups blueberries

½ cup toasted almonds

1 recipe (about 1 cup) Regal Lemon-Shallot Dressing (page 319)

In a large bowl, layer the kale, barley, chickpeas, broccoli, chicken, beets, blueberries, and almonds. Pour the dressing over the salad and toss to combine.

Nutritional analysis per serving (serving size: ¼ salad + ¼ cup dressing): Calories: 425, Total Fat: 14 g, Saturated Fat: 1.5 g, Trans fat: 0 g, Polyunsaturated Fat: 3 g, Mono-unsaturated Fat: 6 g, Cholesterol: 70 mg, Sodium: 500 mg, Total Carbohydrates: 43 g, Dietary Fiber: 10 g, Total Sugars: 8 g (including 0 g added sugar), Protein: 33 g

Turkey Chili

MIND POINTS: 1 SERVING = 1.5 OV, 0.5 POUL, 0.5 BN

Chili is an American classic. Although it varies regionally, one thing we can agree on is that it is delicious, relatively easy to make, and oh so comforting. For those of us who live in colder climates, it is a staple. This version uses ground turkey, green chiles, and yellow squash to lighten up the ingredients but still provides the classic chili taste and texture. My family loves it served over whole-wheat penne or fusilli. I like to top it with a sprinkle of high-quality cheddar cheese. Whatever you choose, this will become a go-to family favorite.

Serves: 7
Prep time: 15 minutes
Cook time: 45 minutes

   1 tablespoon extra-virgin olive oil

   1 pound ground turkey

   1 tablespoon dried oregano

   1 tablespoon ground cumin

   2 teaspoons chili powder

   1 teaspoon garlic powder

   1 teaspoon onion powder

   ¼ teaspoon salt

   2 garlic cloves, chopped

   1 small yellow onion, finely chopped

   2 cups diced yellow squash or zucchini (or corn)

   2 (15-ounce) cans fire-roasted tomatoes

   1 (15-ounce) can black beans, drained and rinsed

   1 (15-ounce) can pinto beans, drained and rinsed

1 (4-ounce) can green chiles (mild or hot), drained

1 cup low-sodium chicken broth, plus 1 cup water

Heat the oil in a large, heavy-bottomed pot over medium heat. Add the turkey and cook until lightly browned and mostly cooked through, 4 to 7 minutes.

Add the oregano, cumin, chili powder, garlic powder, onion powder, and salt. Stir to coat the turkey and cook for another 2 minutes. Transfer the turkey to a bowl.

Add the onion and squash to the pot and cook for 3 to 5 minutes, until slightly tender and lightly browned. Return the turkey to the pot, along with the fire-roasted tomatoes with their juices, black beans, pinto beans, chiles, and broth. Mix well. Turn the heat down to medium-low and cook at a gentle simmer for 20 minutes.

Nutritional analysis per serving (serving size: 2 cups): Calories: 320, Total Fat: 10 g, Saturated Fat: 2 g, Trans fat: 0 g, Polyunsaturated Fat: 2 g, Monounsaturated Fat: 3 g, Cholesterol: 45 mg, Sodium: 490 mg, Total Carbohydrates: 36 g, Dietary Fiber: 8 g, Total Sugars: 5 g (including 0 g added sugar), Protein: 25 g

MIND Diet Board

MIND POINTS: 1 SERVING = 1 LG, 1 OV, 0.5 BER, 0.5 NUT, 0.5 FSH, 0.5 POUL, 0.5 WG

This MIND-diet food board, shown on the cover of this book, is a beautiful, tasty way to feed your guests and loved ones. It can be made using any fresh, vibrant vegetables, and you can customize it to meet all dietary preferences. I often make it for my family for a fun weekend meal.

Serves: 8
Prep time: 25 minutes

1 cup hummus

¼ cup extra-virgin olive oil

¼ cup Pickled Red Onions (page 320)

6 ounces smoked salmon

10 whole-grain crackers

5 small slices whole-grain bread, cut in halves or quarters

3 or 4 skewers Grilled Chicken Spiedies (page 256)

6 small lettuce-leaf cups

2 cups Roasted Kale Chips (page 297)

4 small carrots, peeled and halved lengthwise

3 mini cucumbers, cut into spears

4 mini bell peppers, halved lengthwise and seeded

½ cup sugar snap peas

½ cup blueberries

½ cup blackberries

½ cup sliced strawberries

½ cup raspberries

¼ cup shelled pistachios

¼ cup almonds

¼ cup pumpkin seeds

Grab a large wooden board or decorative serving platter. Put the hummus and oil in small bowls or ramekins. Place these on the board. Top the hummus with the pickled onions. Arrange the smoked salmon around the hummus and oil. Add the crackers and bread.

Add the chicken skewers to the board. Add the lettuce cups and kale chips. Distribute the carrots, cucumbers, peppers, and snap peas so they are evenly dispersed and visually appealing.

Scatter the blueberries, blackberries, strawberries, and raspberries around the board for pops of color. Scatter the pistachios, almonds, and pumpkin seeds, too.

Nutritional analysis per serving (serving size: ⅛ of board): Calories: 450, Total Fat: 27 g, Saturated Fat: 3.5 g, Trans fat: 0 g, Polyunsaturated Fat: 4 g, Monounsaturated Fat: 16 g, Cholesterol: 35 mg, Sodium: 840 mg, Total Carbohydrates: 29 g, Dietary Fiber: 6 g, Total Sugars: 7 g (including 0 g added sugar), Protein: 26 g

Roast Chicken

MIND POINTS: 1 SERVING = 1.5 OV, 2 POUL

A beautiful roast chicken dinner is a classic meal enjoyed throughout the world. It was a meal my father had growing up here in the Midwest, and one he made for us during our childhood, usually on Sunday. This version of roast chicken is just as I remembered his to be—juicy and flavorful. For the tastiest chicken, aim to buy pasture-raised chicken if it is available at your local grocery store. We recommend removing the skin to reduce the amount of saturated fat and sodium. The chicken is just as delicious and juicy with the skin removed. I like to serve a light salad and a seasonal vegetable alongside.

Serves: 6
Prep time: 15 minutes
Cook time: 1 to 1½ hours

    1 (4-pound) chicken

    2 teaspoons salt

    1 lemon, quartered

    6 garlic cloves, peeled

    ½ teaspoon black pepper

    2 medium yellow onions, quartered

    5 large carrots, peeled and cut into large batons

    2 tablespoons avocado oil

265

Preheat the oven to 450°F.

Remove any giblets that may be in the cavity of the chicken and discard. Rinse the chicken under cold water, then dry it well with paper towels, inside and out. Less moisture on the skin results in better browning, which is important for keeping the chicken moist.

Add ¼ teaspoon of the salt to the bird's cavity, then stuff the lemon quarters and garlic cloves inside. Rub the remaining 1¾ teaspoons salt all over the exposed skin, then sprinkle the pepper on top.

Place the chicken breast-side up in a roasting pan. Roast, undisturbed, for 30 minutes.

In a medium bowl, toss the onions and carrots with the avocado oil. Scatter the onions and carrots around the chicken.

Return the pan to the oven and roast for another 30 to 40 minutes. Using a thermometer, check the internal temperature at the thickest part of the thigh and the thickest part of the breast. You want a reading of 165°F to ensure the chicken is cooked through. Return to the oven if more cooking time is needed, and check every 10 minutes.

Transfer the chicken to a cutting board and let rest for 10 to 15 minutes. Reserve all the cooking juices in the pan.

Carve the chicken by first removing the legs and thighs and transferring them to a serving platter. Cut the breast down the middle. Gently remove the skin from the breast, slice the meat on a bias, and transfer to the serving platter. Add the wings to the platter.

Scatter the onions and carrots around the chicken. Spoon the pan juices over the chicken and vegetables.

Nutritional analysis per serving (serving size: 4 ounces chicken + ½ cup veggies): Calories: 410, Total Fat: 13 g, Saturated Fat: 3 g, Trans fat: 0 g, Polyunsaturated Fat: 3 g, Monounsaturated Fat: 6 g, Cholesterol: 195 mg, Sodium: 780 mg, Total Carbohydrates: 8 g, Dietary Fiber: 2 g, Total Sugars: 3 g (including 0 g added sugar), Protein: 62 g

Spaghetti Squash Bolognese

MIND POINTS: 1 SERVING = 0.5 LG, 3 OV, 1 EVOO, 1 POUL

Spaghetti squash is named for its long, sturdy spaghetti-like strands that become tender when cooked. It is delicious on its own and even better when topped with a savory Bolognese sauce. Here we use ground turkey instead of beef. You could also use veggie grounds if you want a vegan option.

Serves: 4
Prep time: 15 minutes
Cook time: 40 minutes

1 spaghetti squash

4 tablespoons extra-virgin olive oil

¼ teaspoon salt

¼ teaspoon black pepper

1 pound ground turkey or veggie grounds

2 cups sliced cremini mushrooms

1 garlic clove, chopped

1 tablespoon balsamic vinegar

½ teaspoon fish sauce

½ teaspoon smoked paprika

2 cups shredded kale

1 (24-ounce) jar tomato sauce

¼ cup grated Parmesan cheese or nutritional yeast (optional)

Preheat the oven to 400°F.

Trim the ends off the squash and cut it in half lengthwise. Scoop out the seeds with a spoon.

Using 2 tablespoons of the oil, lightly oil each squash half and season with the salt and pepper. Place the squash halves cut-side down on a rimmed baking sheet. Bake for 40 minutes, or until a knife inserted into the skin pierces through somewhat easily.

While the squash is cooking, heat 1 tablespoon oil in a large skillet over medium heat. Add the turkey or veggie grounds and sauté, stirring frequently, until just browned, 5 to 8 minutes for turkey or 4 to 6 minutes for veggie grounds. Transfer to a bowl.

Add the remaining 1 tablespoon oil to the pan and heat over medium heat. Add the mushrooms and sauté, stirring occasionally, until they are golden brown, 3 to 5 minutes. Add the garlic and stir just until fragrant, 1 to 2 minutes. Add the balsamic vinegar, fish sauce, and smoked paprika and cook for another 2 minutes. Add the shredded kale and stir just until slightly wilted, about 2 minutes.

Stir in the tomato sauce and ground turkey and let simmer for 3 to 5 minutes. Remove from the heat.

Flip the squash halves cut-side up. Using oven mitts, place on a cutting board and, using two forks, gently scrape the squash to get spaghetti-like strands. Transfer to a serving bowl and top with the Bolognese sauce. Garnish with Parmesan cheese or nutritional yeast, if desired.

Nutritional analysis per serving (serving size: 1½ cups): Calories: 390, Total Fat: 18 g, Saturated Fat: 3 g, Trans fat: 0 g, Polyunsaturated Fat: 2.5 g, Monounsaturated Fat: 11 g, Cholesterol: 60 mg, Sodium: 920 mg, Total Carbohydrates: 26 g, Dietary Fiber: 3 g, Total Sugars: 14 g (including 0 g added sugar), Protein: 32 g

Broiled Arctic Char

MIND POINTS: 1 SERVING = 1 FSH

Broiling fish is an easy technique that is time-efficient and creates a visually appealing finish. A marinade with citrus and oil helps protect the fish from AGEs (advanced glycation end products). Artic char is a cold-water fish that is high in omega-3 fatty acids and has a pink flesh similar to salmon. But instead of Arctic char, you can use another hearty fish like salmon, mahi-mahi, or halibut. We love this over a bed of greens like Arugula Hemp Seed Salad (page 292). It also pairs well with quinoa or brown rice.

Serves: 4
Prep time: 7 minutes, plus 30 minutes to marinate
Cook time: 5 minutes

- 3 tablespoons lime juice
- 2 tablespoons avocado oil
- 2 tablespoons low-sodium soy sauce
- 1 tablespoon honey
- 4 (4-ounce) Arctic char fillets
- ¼ teaspoon salt

In a large, shallow bowl, whisk together the lime juice, oil, soy sauce, and honey. Place the Arctic char fillets flesh-side down in the marinade, cover, and refrigerate for up to 30 minutes.

Place an oven rack 6 to 7 inches from the heating element. Preheat the oven to broil. Lightly grease a rimmed baking sheet with cooking spray or oil.

Transfer the fillets to the prepared baking sheet, skin-side down, and broil for 4 to 7 minutes, depending on the thickness of the fish. You want it to have a slightly golden-brown char and to be cooked through; it should easily flake with a fork.

Remove from the oven and sprinkle with the salt.

Nutritional analysis per serving (serving size: 1 fillet): Calories: 290, Total Fat: 19 g, Saturated Fat: 4 g, Trans fat: 0 g, Polyunsaturated Fat: 4 g, Monounsaturated Fat: 10 g, Cholesterol: 55 mg, Sodium: 455 mg, Total Carbohydrates: 6 g, Dietary Fiber: 0 g, Total Sugars: 5 g (including 0 g added sugar), Protein: 23 g

Poached Salmon with Toasted Almonds and Parsley

MIND POINTS: 1 SERVING = 0.5 EVOO, 1 NUT, 1 FSH

Poaching is a delicious and light cooking technique that can infuse fish with aromatics and flavor, all while keeping it tender and juicy. This recipe uses fresh rosemary and thyme, but you could use any fresh herbs you have on hand. I like using wild-caught king or coho salmon. The toasted almonds and parsley add texture and a balance of flavors that go beautifully with the fish. Serve with a light grain like quinoa or brown rice and a green salad.

Serves: 4
Prep time: 15 minutes
Cook time: 15 minutes

4 (4-ounce) salmon fillets, bones removed

½ teaspoon salt

½ yellow onion, sliced

¾ cup water

½ cup dry white wine

1 or 2 rosemary sprigs

1 or 2 thyme sprigs

¾ cup sliced almonds

1 small shallot, finely chopped

1 cup chopped fresh parsley

2 tablespoons red wine vinegar

2 tablespoons extra-virgin olive oil

Sprinkle the salmon with ¼ teaspoon of the salt; set aside.

In a large skillet, combine the onion, water, wine, and herb sprigs. Cover and bring to a light simmer over medium heat. Add the salmon to the pan (skin-side down if your salmon has skin), cover, and cook at a light simmer for 10 to 12 minutes, until the salmon is cooked through. You can test by lightly flaking the middle of the salmon with a fork. Remove the pan from the heat.

While the salmon is cooking, put the sliced almonds in a small saucepan and toast over medium heat, stirring every 60 to 90 seconds, until the almonds are lightly golden, 3 to 4 minutes. Transfer the almonds to a bowl. Add the shallot, parsley, vinegar, oil, and remaining ¼ teaspoon salt. Mix until well combined.

Transfer the salmon to a serving dish, discarding the poaching liquid, onion, and herb sprigs. Top with the parsley and almond mixture.

Nutritional analysis per serving (serving size: 1 fillet): Calories: 370, Total Fat: 26 g, Saturated Fat: 3 g, Trans fat: 0 g, Polyunsaturated Fat: 6 g, Monounsaturated Fat: 15 g, Cholesterol: 60 mg, Sodium: 350 mg, Total Carbohydrates: 7 g, Dietary Fiber: 4 g, Total Sugars: 2 g (including 0 g added sugar), Protein: 28 g

Pasta with Marinated Tomatoes and Shrimp

MIND POINTS: 1 SERVING = 1 OV, 1 EVOO, 1 FSH, 2 WG

I love a simple, elegant pasta dish that is no fuss in the kitchen. This dish calls for shrimp, but it is just as delicious on its own as a vegetarian dinner. Whole-wheat spaghetti is easy to find in most grocery stores now, or you could try other options, like rice, lentil, or quinoa spaghetti. This dish is delicious served warm or chilled.

Serves: 6
Prep time: 10 minutes, plus 2 hours to marinate
Cook time: 10 minutes

2 pints cherry tomatoes, halved

¼ cup plus 1 tablespoon extra-virgin olive oil

1 large shallot, thinly sliced

3 garlic cloves, chopped

2 teaspoons grated lemon zest

⅓ cup lemon juice

½ teaspoon salt

½ teaspoon black pepper

1 pound whole-wheat spaghetti

1½ pounds large shrimp, peeled and deveined

⅓ cup chopped fresh basil or parsley

In a large bowl, combine the tomatoes, ¼ cup of the oil, the shallot, garlic, lemon zest, lemon juice, salt, and pepper. Let marinate for 2 hours at room temperature.

Bring a large pot of salted water to a boil. Add the spaghetti and cook for 8 minutes, or until al dente. Drain. Add the spaghetti to the tomato mixture and toss.

While the pasta is cooking, heat the remaining 1 tablespoon oil in a large skillet over medium-high heat. Pat the shrimp dry and add them to the pan in a single layer, working in batches as necessary so you don't crowd the pan. Cook for 1 to 1½ minutes for a light sear. Flip and cook for 30 to 60 seconds on the other side, until the shrimp is just cooked through.

Add the shrimp to the spaghetti. Gently stir to combine all the ingredients. Top with fresh basil or parsley just before serving.

Nutritional analysis per serving (serving size: 1½ cups): Calories: 530, Total Fat: 20 g, Saturated Fat: 3 g, Trans fat: 0 g, Polyunsaturated Fat: 3 g, Monounsaturated Fat: 14 g, Cholesterol: 145 mg, Sodium: 870 mg, Total Carbohydrates: 64 g, Dietary Fiber: 8 g, Total Sugars: 4 g (including 0 g added sugar), Protein: 27 g

Chickpea Tuna Salad

MIND POINTS: 1 SERVING = 0.5 OV, 1 EVOO, 0.5 FSH, 0.5 BN

For those of you who love a lot of texture and bite in your food, this is for you! This salad is an easy, colorful, and protein-packed lunch or light dinner that comes together quickly. You can use any fresh herb you like, and dried herbs work as well. This dish is great on its own or over a bed of whatever fresh leafy greens you have on hand. You can also serve it with your favorite whole-grain toast.

Serves: 4
Prep time: 10 minutes

    1 (15-ounce) can chickpeas, drained and rinsed

    1 (6-ounce) can tuna, drained

    3 cups shredded carrots

    ½ cup chopped fresh parsley

    Juice of 1 lemon

    Juice of 1 orange

    ¼ cup extra-virgin olive oil

    1 teaspoon toasted sesame oil

    ¼ teaspoon ground cumin

    ¼ teaspoon salt

In a large bowl, combine the chickpeas, tuna, carrots, and parsley.

In a small bowl, whisk together the lemon juice, orange juice, olive oil, sesame oil, cumin, and salt. Pour the dressing over the chickpeas and tuna and toss gently until well combined.

Nutritional analysis per serving (serving size: 1 cup): Calories: 280, Total Fat: 17 g, Saturated Fat: 2.5 g, Trans fat: 0 g, Polyunsaturated Fat: 2 g, Monounsaturated Fat: 11 g, Cholesterol: 15 mg, Sodium: 440 mg, Total Carbohydrates: 21 g, Dietary Fiber: 5 g, Total Sugars: 6 g (including 0 g added sugar), Protein: 13 g

Lentil Quinoa Salad with Smoked Salmon

MIND POINTS: 1 SERVING = 1 OV, 1 EVOO, 0.5 FSH, 1 WG, 1 BN

This filling and nutrient-packed grain salad is a great make-ahead meal for grab-and-go lunches. The light quinoa combined with the meatier lentils is a great balance of textures. You can keep this salad vegan by omitting the salmon and adding pine nuts or any other nut you prefer. The salad has a light vinaigrette, but you could use any favorite salad dressing you have on hand. Even a little EVOO and lemon juice works great!

Serves: 6
Prep time: 15 minutes
Cook time: 25 minutes

1 cup green lentils

1 cup quinoa

2 cups low-sodium vegetable broth

¼ teaspoon salt

2 cups diced cucumber

2 cups halved cherry or grape tomatoes

1 cup pitted kalamata olives, halved

12 ounces smoked salmon, broken into pieces

⅓ cup chopped fresh parsley

¼ cup plus 2 tablespoons extra-virgin olive oil

Juice of 1 small lemon

2 tablespoons apple cider vinegar

1 tablespoon pure maple syrup

Put the lentils in a fine-mesh strainer and rinse under cold running water for about 2 minutes. Discard any pebbles or other debris that may be present. Put the lentils in a medium saucepan and pour in enough water to cover them by about 2 inches. Bring to a boil over medium-high heat, then reduce to a simmer, cover, and cook for 15 to 20 minutes, until the lentils are cooked through and slightly tender. Drain.

Meanwhile, put the quinoa in the fine-mesh strainer and rinse under cold running water for at least 2 minutes. In another medium saucepan, combine the quinoa, broth, and salt. Bring to a boil over medium-high heat, then reduce to a simmer, cover, and cook for 10 minutes, until the quinoa is plump and tender. Remove from the heat and let sit for 5 minutes, covered, then fluff with a fork.

In a large bowl, combine the lentils and quinoa. Add the cucumber, tomatoes, olives, salmon, and parsley.

In a small bowl, whisk together the oil, lemon juice, vinegar, and maple syrup. Pour the dressing over the salad and toss to combine.

Nutritional analysis per serving (serving size: 1 cup): Calories: 400, Total Fat: 19 g, Saturated Fat: 3 g, Trans fat: 0 g, Polyunsaturated Fat: 3 g, Monounsaturated Fat: 12 g, Cholesterol: 15 mg, Sodium: 690 mg, Total Carbohydrates: 39 g, Dietary Fiber: 9 g, Total Sugars: 3 g (including 0 g added sugar), Protein: 21 g

White Fish with Olives and Artichokes

MIND POINTS: 1 SERVING = 1 OV, 1 EVOO, 1 FSH

There are many varieties of white-fleshed fish—sole, tilapia, cod, halibut, snapper, bass, to name a few! These fish all have slightly different textures while all being mild in flavor. This recipe calls for Chilean sea bass, but any white fish will work. Just be sure to adjust the cooking time as needed—the thicker the fish, the longer the cooking time. No matter which fish you choose, this dish bursts with flavor and can be made in less than 30 minutes. Remember to pat your fish with a paper towel to remove excess moisture; this is key to forming a nice crust and preventing the fish from sticking to the pan. I love serving this meal with angel hair pasta and salad.

Serves: 4
Prep time: 10 minutes
Cook time: 20 minutes

   4 (4-ounce) Chilean sea bass fillets or white fish of choice

   ¼ teaspoon salt

   ¼ teaspoon black pepper

   1 tablespoon plus ⅓ cup extra-virgin olive oil

   1 cup pitted Castelvetrano green olives

   1 (12-ounce) jar marinated artichoke hearts, drained

   4 garlic cloves, sliced

   1 lemon, quartered

   2 thyme sprigs

   1 rosemary sprig

   4 ounces light feta cheese, crumbled (optional)

   Pinch crushed red pepper (optional)

Pat the fish dry with a paper towel. Season both sides with the salt and pepper.

Heat 1 tablespoon of the oil in a large skillet over medium-high heat. Add the fish and cook until browned on both sides but not quite cooked through, 3 to 7 minutes per side depending on the thickness and type of fish.

Turn the heat down to medium and add the olives, artichoke hearts, and garlic. Stir to incorporate around the fish. Add the remaining ⅓ cup oil, lemon quarters, and herb sprigs. Using tongs, gently press the lemon and herbs into the pan to add flavor.

Turn the heat down to medium-low, partially cover the pan, and cook for 5 to 7 minutes, until the fish gently flakes when pressed in the center with a fork. You can remove the herb sprigs or use them as a garnish to decorate the plate.

Carefully transfer the fish to a serving platter. Spoon the artichoke and olive mixture around the fish. Drizzle any sauce remaining in the pan on top. Garnish with the feta cheese and crushed red pepper, if desired.

Nutritional analysis per serving (serving size: 1 fillet + ½ cup veggies): Calories: 360, Total Fat: 24 g, Saturated Fat: 4 g, Trans fat: 0 g, Polyunsaturated Fat: 3 g, Monoun- saturated Fat: 16 g, Cholesterol: 45 mg, Sodium: 720 mg, Total Carbohydrates: 14 g, Dietary Fiber: 9 g, Total Sugars: 1 g (including 0 g added sugar), Protein: 24 g

Black Bean Veggie Burgers

MIND POINTS: 1 SERVING = 0.5 BN

These black bean burgers are delicious and crowd-pleasing. Veggie burgers are also the perfect way to use up old veggies and leftover grains and beans. This is a great prep-ahead meal, because the burgers benefit from some time in the refrigerator or freezer before you cook them. The colder they are, the less likely they are to crumble while cooking. As with most burgers, it's the toppings that make them. Feel free to top these with pickles, lettuce, tomato slices, avocado slices, or fresh or Pickled Red Onions (page 320). They're great on whole-wheat buns or with a leafy green salad.

Serves: 8
Prep time: 30 minutes, plus 1 hour to chill
Cook time: 25 minutes

3 tablespoons extra-virgin olive oil

½ small yellow onion, finely chopped

2 garlic cloves, minced

1 small red bell pepper, seeded and cut into small dice

1 small zucchini, cut into small dice

1½ teaspoons ground cumin

1 teaspoon smoked paprika

1 teaspoon onion powder

1 teaspoon salt

½ teaspoon chili powder

2 (15-ounce) cans black beans, drained and rinsed, or 3 cups
   cooked black beans

½ cup cooked brown rice or quinoa

½ cup whole-wheat or panko bread crumbs

⅓ cup chopped fresh cilantro or parsley

Heat 1 tablespoon of the oil in a large skillet over medium heat. Add the onion and sauté until translucent, 1 to 2 minutes. Add the garlic, bell pepper, and zucchini and cook for 3 to 4 minutes, until the vegetables are tender. Stir in the cumin, paprika, onion powder, salt, and chili powder and cook for 2 minutes.

Add the black beans and remove the pan from the heat. Using a masher or large fork, mash well until most of the black beans are smashed, leaving some intact. Transfer to a large bowl and stir in the cooked rice and bread crumbs.

Let cool for 10 minutes, then cover and transfer to the refrigerator for at least 30 minutes.

Mix in the cilantro and form into 8 patties. Return to the refrigerator for at least 20 minutes or up to overnight to let the burgers set. The colder the patties, the better they will hold their shape while cooking.

Heat 1 tablespoon of the oil in a large skillet over medium heat. Add 4 patties and cook for 2 to 4 minutes, until lightly golden brown. Flip and cook on the other side. Transfer to a plate. Add the remaining 1 tablespoon oil and cook the remaining 4 patties in the same way.

Nutritional analysis per serving (serving size: 1 burger): Calories: 180, Total Fat: 6 g, Saturated Fat: 1 g, Trans fat: 0 g, Polyunsaturated Fat: 0.5 g, Monounsaturated Fat: 4 g, Cholesterol: 0 mg, Sodium: 430 mg, Total Carbohydrates: 24 g, Dietary Fiber: 7 g, Total Sugars: 2 g (including 0 g added sugar), Protein: 7 g

Carrot, Ginger, and Leek Soup

MIND POINTS: 1 SERVING = 2 OV

This recipe is from my husband's granny. She is Hungarian and everything this soup is—bright, colorful, spicy, and nourishing. I made a few adjustments to make it just as delicious but more brain-healthy. We like to serve it with homemade croutons and a colorful salad.

Serves: 6
Prep time: 30 minutes
Cook time: 30 minutes

    2 tablespoons extra-virgin olive oil

    6 large carrots, chopped (about 4 cups)

    1 leek (white part only), chopped

    1 russet potato, peeled and chopped (about 1½ cups)

    1 medium yellow onion, chopped

    ½ teaspoon salt

    1 tablespoon grated fresh ginger

    2½ cups low-sodium vegetable broth

    1½ cups milk of choice

    Hot sauce (optional)

Heat the oil in a medium saucepan over medium heat. Add the carrots, leek, potato, onion, and salt and cook, stirring frequently, until the carrots are bright and slightly tender, about 7 minutes. Stir in the ginger.

Add the broth and bring to a boil. Reduce the heat to medium-low, cover, and simmer for 20 minutes, or until the veggies are soft and cooked through.

Using a hand blender, carefully puree until smooth and creamy. Return to medium-low heat and stir in the milk. Bring back to a light simmer. Ladle into bowls and add a couple drops of hot sauce to each serving, if desired.

Nutritional analysis per serving (serving size: 1 cup): Calories: 180, Total Fat: 7 g, Saturated Fat: 1 g, Trans fat: 0 g, Polyunsaturated Fat: 0.5 g, Monounsaturated Fat: 3.5 g, Cholesterol: 0 mg, Sodium: 640 mg, Total Carbohydrates: 28 g, Dietary Fiber: 5 g, Total Sugars: 9 g (including 2 g added sugar), Protein: 3 g

Rice Noodles with Stir-Fried Vegetables

MIND POINTS: 1 SERVING = 0.5 LG, 2.5 OV, 1 WG

If there is a dish that can be both light and hearty at the same time, this is it. The sauce is oh so light while also loaded with flavor. I love this dish when I am really wanting a big dose of vegetables. Whenever I make a stir-fry, I like to prep all my ingredients and sauces before I begin to cook. That way I can just grab and toss in for a quick meal that comes together effortlessly. This recipe has edamame and peanuts, but you could also add chicken or shrimp for extra protein.

Serves: 8
Prep time: 20 minutes
Cook time: 20 minutes

Stir-Fry:

    1 (16-ounce) package brown rice noodles

    2 tablespoons extra-virgin olive oil

    2 cups sliced shiitake mushrooms

2 large carrots, peeled and cut into matchsticks

1 head broccoli, cut into bite-size pieces

⅓ water (optional)

2 cups shredded kale

Sauce:

½ cup orange juice

3 tablespoons coconut aminos *or* 1½ teaspoons low-sodium soy
sauce plus 1 teaspoon honey

2 tablespoons low-sodium soy sauce

1 tablespoon rice wine vinegar

2 teaspoons toasted sesame oil

1 tablespoon minced fresh ginger or ginger paste

2 garlic cloves, chopped

Garnish:

⅔ cup frozen edamame, cooked according to package instructions

⅓ cup roasted peanuts, roughly chopped

3 tablespoons roughly chopped fresh cilantro

Cook the rice noodles according to the package instructions, then
drain and rinse under cold water to remove excess starch so they don't
clump together.

Meanwhile, heat 1 tablespoon of the olive oil in a large skillet
over medium-high heat. Add the mushrooms and sauté, stirring
occasionally, until lightly golden brown, 3 to 5 minutes. Transfer to a
medium bowl.

Add the remaining 1 tablespoon olive oil to the pan. When hot, add
the carrots and broccoli and sauté for 5 to 7 minutes, until the veggies
are bright and slightly tender but still crisp. Add the water and cover
the pan if you want your veggies a bit more fork-tender.

Stir in the kale and cook until just slightly wilted but still bright green, about 2 minutes. Transfer the veggies to the bowl with the mushrooms.

In a medium bowl, whisk together all the sauce ingredients.

Transfer the noodles to the same skillet and set over medium-low heat. Add the sauce and gently mix to coat the noodles and lightly cook the garlic and ginger in the sauce, 2 to 3 minutes.

Transfer the noodles to a serving bowl, add the veggies, and toss. Top with the edamame, peanuts, and cilantro.

Nutritional analysis per serving (serving size: 1 cup): Calories: 340, Total Fat: 10 g, Saturated Fat: 2 g, Trans fat: 0 g, Polyunsaturated Fat: 1.5 g, Monounsaturated Fat: 5 g, Cholesterol: 0 mg, Sodium: 400 mg, Total Carbohydrates: 55 g, Dietary Fiber: 2 g, Total Sugars: 6 g (including 0 g added sugar), Protein: 9 g

Crispy Fried Rice

MIND POINTS: 1 SERVING = 1 LG, 1.5 OV, 0.5 EVOO, 1 WG

Growing up, we would have stir-fried brown rice at least once a week. It is a great way to use up leftover rice and an easy meal to throw together. You can use almost any vegetables you have on hand. I love the contrasting textures of the crispy rice, softer vegetables, and creamy avocado. Add garlic, olive oil, and some of your favorite seasonings, and you have a delicious meal ready to go. This recipe is vegan, but you can always add any protein you have on hand or top with a fried egg.

Serves: 6
Prep time: 10 minutes
Cook time: 40 minutes

2 tablespoons extra-virgin olive oil, or more as needed
2 teaspoons toasted sesame oil

1 large or 2 small sweet potatoes, peeled and cut into bite-size
   pieces

1 tablespoon Old Bay Seasoning

2 cups sliced cremini mushrooms

1 bunch kale, stemmed and cut into 1-inch pieces

1 garlic clove, chopped

1 tablespoon chopped fresh ginger

2 tablespoons coconut aminos *or* 1 tablespoon low-sodium soy
   sauce plus 1 teaspoon honey

3 cups cooked brown rice

1 avocado, peeled, pitted, and sliced

½ cup chopped scallions

In a large skillet, heat 1 tablespoon of the olive oil and 1 teaspoon of
the sesame oil over medium heat. Add the sweet potatoes and sauté,
stirring frequently, for 3 to 4 minutes. Add the Old Bay and cook for
another 5 minutes, or until the sweet potatoes are slightly golden and
cooked through. Transfer to a bowl.

Add the mushrooms to the pan and sauté for 3 to 4 minutes,
stirring occasionally, until just browned. You can add a little more olive
oil if the pan seems dry.

Add the kale and stir, allowing the leaves to wilt and turn bright
green, about 2 minutes. Return the sweet potatoes to the pan, along
with the garlic and ginger. Sauté for 2 minutes. Add the coconut
aminos and stir to incorporate. Transfer to the same bowl.

Add the remaining 1 tablespoon olive oil and 1 teaspoon sesame
oil to the pan. When hot, add the rice and spread it out so it covers the
bottom of the pan. Do not stir; let it cook for 2 minutes to get a slight
crunch.

Using a wooden spoon, scrape the rice from the bottom and mix.
Let cook for another 2 minutes without stirring. Repeat once or twice
more to create layers of crispy, golden brown rice.

Return the veggies to the pan and gently toss to combine all ingredients. Top with the avocado slices and chopped scallions.

Nutritional analysis per serving (serving size: 1 cup): Calories: 280, Total Fat: 11 g, Saturated Fat: 1.5 g, Trans fat: 0 g, Polyunsaturated Fat: 1 g, Monounsaturated Fat: 6 g, Cholesterol: 0 mg, Sodium: 540 mg, Total Carbohydrates: 41 g, Dietary Fiber: 5 g, Total Sugars: 4 g (including 0 g added sugar), Protein: 6 g

Curried Coconut Vegetable Stew

MIND POINTS: 1 SERVING = 0.5 LG, 1 OV, 0.5 EVOO

This is one of my favorite plant-based dishes to make. It is hearty comfort food, full of brain-healthy vegetables, and it fills the kitchen with the most delicious fragrance. Canned coconut milk can be high in saturated fat, so be sure to buy the light version. Serve this over brown rice, wild rice, or warm toasted naan bread.

Serves: 8
Prep time: 15 minutes
Cook time: 15 minutes

4 tablespoons extra-virgin olive oil

1 small yellow onion, diced

3 garlic cloves, chopped

1 tablespoon chopped fresh ginger

1 tablespoon garam masala

1 tablespoon Old Bay Seasoning

1 tablespoon curry powder

⅓ cup dry white wine

1 sweet potato, peeled and cut into small dice

2 cups sliced cremini mushrooms

1 (15-ounce) can chickpeas, drained and rinsed

¼ teaspoon salt

2 cups low-sodium vegetable broth

1 (15-ounce) can light coconut milk

4 cups roughly chopped kale

Juice of 1 lime

2 to 3 tablespoons chopped fresh cilantro

Heat 2 tablespoons of the oil in a large saucepan over medium heat. Add the onion, garlic, and ginger and cook, stirring frequently, until the onion is almost translucent, about 3 minutes. Add the garam masala, Old Bay, and curry powder and stir to coat the onion. Stir in the white wine to deglaze the pan and let it simmer for 2 to 3 minutes.

Add the remaining 2 tablespoons oil, sweet potato, mushrooms, chickpeas, and salt. Lightly stir and then add the broth. Bring to a light simmer and cook until the sweet potato is fork-tender, about 8 minutes.

Reduce the heat to low and add the coconut milk and kale. Stir until the kale is just wilted, about 2 minutes. Remove from the heat and add the lime juice and cilantro.

Nutritional analysis per serving (serving size: 1 cup): Calories: 200, Total Fat: 10 g, Saturated Fat: 3 g, Trans fat: 0 g, Polyunsaturated Fat: 1 g, Monounsaturated Fat: 6 g, Cholesterol: 0 mg, Sodium: 570 mg, Total Carbohydrates: 22 g, Dietary Fiber: 5 g, Total Sugars: 5 g (including 0 g added sugar), Protein: 6 g

Warm Veggie Wrap

MIND POINTS: 1 SERVING = 1 LG, 2.5 OV, 1 EVOO, 1 WG, 1 BN

We love a good wrap for a light dinner or veggie-packed lunch. This recipe uses Mediterranean-inspired flavors to really elevate the meal.

Add any veggies you have on hand, like bell peppers and tomatoes. Be sure to use a tortilla wrap big enough to hold all the filling. These wraps are vegetarian, but you could always add chicken (or tofu) to boost the protein.

Serves: 2
Prep time: 10 minutes
Cook time: 10 minutes

- 2 tablespoons extra-virgin olive oil
- 2 cups sliced cremini mushrooms
- 1 cup diced zucchini
- 1 garlic clove, chopped
- 2 cups chopped kale
- 2 medium or large whole-grain tortilla wraps
- 4 tablespoons hummus
- ¼ cup halved kalamata olives

Heat the oil in a large skillet over medium heat. Working in batches so you don't crowd the pan, add the mushrooms in a single layer and sauté, stirring occasionally, till the mushrooms have browned, about 2 minutes per side. Transfer to a bowl.

Add the zucchini to the pan and sauté for 2 to 4 minutes, stirring frequently. Add the garlic and kale and sauté until the kale is just wilted, about 2 minutes. Remove the pan from the heat.

Heat the tortilla wraps in a dry skillet for 20 to 30 seconds on each side or in the microwave for 30 seconds, or until warmed.

Spread 2 tablespoons hummus on each tortilla. Spoon about 1 cup veggies on top of the hummus in the center of the wrap. Top with the olives and roll up into wraps. If you have extra veggies, enjoy as a side!

Nutritional analysis per serving (serving size: 1 wrap): Calories: 340, Total Fat: 22 g, Saturated Fat: 3.5 g, Trans fat: 0 g, Polyunsaturated Fat: 2.5 g, Monounsaturated Fat: 12 g, Cholesterol: 0 mg, Sodium: 510 mg, Total Carbohydrates: 32 g, Dietary Fiber: 1 g, Total Sugars: 2 g (including 0 g added sugar), Protein: 9 g

CHAPTER 22

Sides, Salads, and Snacks

Crispy Brussels Sprouts with Savory Sauce

MIND POINTS: 1 SERVING = 1 OV

I love brussels sprouts! They are in the antioxidant-rich family of cruciferous vegetables and can be eaten raw, steamed, roasted, sautéed—you name it. The tangy sauce is so good, you can also use it on seafood, fish, or any other vegetables. I often make a double batch to have in the refrigerator so that I can spruce up almost any meal.

Serves: 6
Prep time: 10 minutes
Cook time: 15 minutes

- 1 pound brussels sprouts, trimmed and halved (or quartered if large)
- 2 tablespoons extra-virgin olive oil
- ¼ teaspoon salt
- ¼ cup coconut aminos *or* 3 tablespoons low-sodium soy sauce plus 1 tablespoon honey
- 3 tablespoons tahini
- 1 tablespoon Dijon mustard
- 1 teaspoon fish sauce

1 teaspoon toasted sesame oil

1 garlic clove, chopped

¼ cup peanuts, roughly chopped

Preheat the oven to 400°F. Line a rimmed baking sheet with aluminum foil.

Put the brussels sprouts on the prepared baking sheet and drizzle with the olive oil and salt. Use your hands to coat all pieces evenly, then arrange them in a single layer, cut-side down. Roast for 15 minutes, or until they are golden brown and slightly crispy.

In a small bowl, whisk together the coconut aminos, tahini, mustard, fish sauce, sesame oil, and garlic.

Transfer the brussels sprouts to a medium bowl. Pour the sauce over them and mix gently to coat. Top with the chopped peanuts.

Nutritional analysis per serving (serving size: ½ cup): Calories: 170, Total Fat: 13 g, Saturated Fat: 2 g, Trans fat: 0 g, Polyunsaturated Fat: 3 g, Monounsaturated Fat: 7 g, Cholesterol: 0 mg, Sodium: 440 mg, Total Carbohydrates: 12 g, Dietary Fiber: 4 g, Total Sugars: 4 g (including 0 g added sugar), Protein: 5 g

Savory Almond Corn on the Cob

MIND POINTS: 1 SERVING = 1 OV, 0.5 NUT

This recipe is inspired by elote corn, a traditional Mexican dish that is served with mayonnaise, lime juice, and cheese. This hits all the same notes but substitutes almonds for the higher-saturated-fat cheese. You can also make it into a dip by cutting the corn off the cob (or using 2 cups thawed frozen corn) and mixing in the sauce and almonds. I like to serve this with Broiled Arctic Char (page 268) or Grilled Chicken Spiedies (page 256).

Serves: 4
Prep time: 5 minutes
Cook time: 15 minutes

- 4 ears corn, husks and silk removed
- ¼ cup mayonnaise
- 1½ tablespoons low-sodium soy sauce
- Grated zest and juice of 1 lime
- ½ teaspoon chili powder
- ¾ cup raw almonds
- ¼ teaspoon salt
- 2 tablespoons chopped fresh cilantro

Preheat a grill or stovetop grill pan over high heat. Grill the corn, turning occasionally, until it is slightly charred and bright yellow, 5 to 7 minutes. (Alternatively, you can pour 2 or 3 inches of water into a large pot and bring to a simmer. Add the corn, cover, and steam until bright yellow and tender, about 5 minutes.)

In a small bowl, mix the mayonnaise, soy sauce, lime zest and juice, and chili powder.

Pulse the almonds and salt in a food processor until they have a sand-like consistency, with some small chunks. Spread out on a plate.

Using a pastry brush or spoon, coat each ear of corn in the mayonnaise mixture, then roll the corn in the almonds to fully coat. Top with the cilantro.

Nutritional analysis per serving (serving size: 1 ear corn): Calories: 240, Total Fat: 16 g, Saturated Fat: 1.5 g, Trans fat: 0 g, Polyunsaturated Fat: 0.5 g, Monounsaturated Fat: 0 g, Cholesterol: 0 mg, Sodium: 250 mg, Total Carbohydrates: 21 g, Dietary Fiber: 4 g, Total Sugars: 3 g (including 0 g added sugar), Protein: 6 g

Sautéed Greens

MIND POINTS: 1 SERVING = 1 LG, 0.5 EVOO

A simple side dish of sautéed greens is a perfect way to get in a hearty dose of your leafy green vegetables. I love having a bowl of these after I have been traveling and haven't been eating well. Swiss chard and Tuscan kale are good options. This dish goes well served with Broiled Arctic Char (page 268), tossed into spaghetti, or mixed with your favorite grains, such as brown rice, farro, or quinoa.

Serves: 6
Prep time: 5 minutes
Cook time: 5 minutes

3 tablespoons extra-virgin olive oil

1 small shallot, chopped

1 bunch rainbow Swiss chard or Tuscan kale, leaves and stems cut into ½-inch pieces (about 5 cups)

1 garlic clove, chopped

¼ teaspoon salt

Heat the oil in a medium skillet over medium-low heat. Add the shallot and cook until translucent, 2 to 3 minutes. Add the Swiss chard and sauté for 2 to 3 minutes, until just slightly wilted. Add the garlic and sauté for another minute. Season with the salt.

Nutritional analysis per serving (serving size: ½ cup): Calories: 60, Total Fat: 4.5 g, Saturated Fat: 0.5 g, Trans fat: 0 g, Polyunsaturated Fat: 0 g, Monounsaturated Fat: 3.5 g, Cholesterol: 0 mg, Sodium: 250 mg, Total Carbohydrates: 5 g, Dietary Fiber: 2 g, Total Sugars: 1 g (including 0 g added sugar), Protein: 2 g

Autumn Roasted Vegetables with Apple Cider Sauce

MIND POINTS: 1 SERVING = 1.5 OV, 0.5 EVOO

There is nothing quite like roasted vegetables, especially when the weather starts to turn slightly crisp and cool. And you can roast almost any vegetable there is! Make this recipe your own by using any vegetables you have on hand—broccoli, cauliflower, squash, carrots, beets, turnips, bell peppers...the list goes on. Just be sure to cut the vegetables in a uniform size and shape for even cooking. This is a great side dish with Roast Chicken (page 265) or Broiled Artic Char (page 268). It's also delicious over a bed of whole grains such as brown rice, farro, or quinoa; spice it up by adding some dried cranberries and crumbled feta or goat cheese.

Serves: 4
Prep time: 20 minutes
Cook time: 30 minutes

3 cups brussels sprouts, trimmed and halved

2 medium carrots, cut on a bias into ½-inch-thick slices

1 medium red onion, cut into ¼-inch-thick slices

2 red bell peppers, seeded and cut into 1-inch pieces

3 tablespoons extra-virgin olive oil

2 tablespoons apple cider or apple juice

1 tablespoon apple cider vinegar

½ teaspoon ground cinnamon

½ teaspoon salt

¼ teaspoon black pepper

1 tablespoon chopped fresh thyme or rosemary (optional)

Preheat the oven to 400°F.

In a large bowl, toss the brussels sprouts, carrots, onion, and bell peppers with 1 tablespoon of the oil. Spread the veggies on a rimmed baking sheet, making sure they are not crowded; use two baking sheets, if necessary. Roast for 20 minutes.

In a small bowl, whisk together the remaining 2 tablespoons oil, apple cider, vinegar, cinnamon, salt, and pepper.

Remove the pan from the oven and add the sauce and fresh herb, if desired. Using a wooden spoon, gently stir the veggies, then return to the oven for another 10 minutes, or until fork-tender.

Nutritional analysis per serving (serving size: 1 cup): Calories: 160, Total Fat: 11 g, Saturated Fat: 1.5 g, Trans fat: 0 g, Polyunsaturated Fat: 1 g, Monounsaturated Fat: 7 g, Cholesterol: 0 mg, Sodium: 330 mg, Total Carbohydrates: 16 g, Dietary Fiber: 5 g, Total Sugars: 7 g (including 0 g added sugar), Protein: 3 g

Arugula Hemp Seed Salad

MIND POINTS: 1 SERVING = 1 LG, 1 EVOO, 1 NUT

This wonderfully simple, elegant salad comes together quickly. The mix of bitter and peppery notes from the arugula and sweet hints from the balsamic reduction is a great balance of flavors. Hemp seeds add healthy fats along with a nutty texture. The salad is a great side to a beautiful piece of salmon, or you could add your favorite vegetables and a sprinkle of nuts to make it into a light lunch. I love to top it with Pickled Red Onions (page 320) to balance out the bitter arugula greens.

Serves: 4
Prep time: 10 minutes
Cook time: 5 minutes

⅔ cup hemp seeds

6 cups arugula

¼ cup extra-virgin olive oil

2 tablespoons Balsamic Reduction (page 317)

¼ teaspoon salt

¼ teaspoon black pepper

Toast the hemp seeds in a medium skillet over medium heat, gently tossing, until golden brown and slightly fragrant, 2 to 3 minutes. Transfer the seeds to a bowl and let cool for 1 to 2 minutes.

Put the arugula in a salad bowl. Drizzle with the oil and balsamic reduction and toss gently. Top with the hemp seeds and toss to combine. Season with the salt and pepper.

Nutritional analysis per serving (serving size: 1¼ cups): Calories: 280, Total Fat: 27 g, Saturated Fat: 3 g, Trans fat: 0 g, Polyunsaturated Fat: 12 g, Monounsaturated Fat: 12 g, Cholesterol: 0 mg, Sodium: 150 mg, Total Carbohydrates: 4 g, Dietary Fiber: 2 g, Total Sugars: 2 g (including 0 g added sugar), Protein: 9 g

Tuscan Kale Salad

MIND POINTS: 1 SERVING = 1 LG, 0.5 BER, 1 EVOO, 0.5 NUT

Tuscan kale, also known as lacinato kale, black kale, or dinosaur kale, has long dark green leaves and is slightly sweeter and more tender than curly kale. I love pairing it with Dijon vinaigrette. Topped with almonds and blueberries, this is a MIND diet super meal! You can eat it as a simple side salad, or add smoked salmon, hard-boiled eggs, tuna, or your protein of choice.

Serves: 4
Prep time: 10 minutes
Cook time: 5 minutes

½ cup slivered almonds

1 bunch Tuscan kale, stems removed, leaves cut into 1-inch pieces

1 cup blueberries

¼ cup extra-virgin olive oil

2 tablespoons apple cider vinegar

2 teaspoons Dijon mustard

¼ teaspoon salt

Lightly toast the almonds in a medium skillet over medium heat, gently stirring, until the nuts turn light golden brown, about 4 minutes. Transfer to a large bowl to cool for 1 to 2 minutes.

Add the kale and blueberries to the bowl with the almonds.

In a small bowl, whisk together the oil, vinegar, mustard, and salt. Drizzle the dressing over the salad and toss to combine.

Nutritional analysis per serving (serving size: 1 cup): Calories: 150, Total Fat: 14 g, Saturated Fat: 2 g, Trans fat: 0 g, Polyunsaturated Fat: 2 g, Monounsaturated Fat: 10 g, Cholesterol: 0 mg, Sodium: 180 mg, Total Carbohydrates: 7 g, Dietary Fiber: 2 g, Total Sugars: 4 g (including 0 g added sugar), Protein: 1 g

Farro and Arugula Salad

MIND POINTS: 1 SERVING = 1 LG, 1 EVOO, 1 WG

Farro is a delicious, nutty, hearty grain that is high in B vitamins, protein, and fiber. I love to make a big batch to throw into soups or to use in a big grain salad like this one. You can customize this salad by adding your favorite chopped veggies. This is a great meal to make for quick, filling lunches that travel well.

Serves: 4
Prep time: 10 minutes
Cook time: 30 minutes

1 cup farro

3 cups low-sodium vegetable broth or water

⅓ cup extra-virgin olive oil

3 tablespoons apple cider vinegar

2 teaspoons honey

¼ teaspoon salt

4 cups arugula

1 green apple, cored and diced

¼ cup shelled pistachios

¼ cup dried cranberries

4 ounces feta cheese, crumbled (optional)

In a medium saucepan, combine the farro and broth. Bring to a boil, then reduce the heat to a simmer, cover, and cook for 20 to 30 minutes, until the farro is tender. Drain any excess liquid and let cool.

In a small bowl, whisk together the oil, vinegar, honey, and salt.

In a large bowl, combine the farro, arugula, apple, pistachios, and cranberries. Toss with the dressing until well combined. Top with the feta cheese, if desired.

Nutritional analysis per serving (serving size: ¼ salad): Calories: 460, Total Fat: 24 g, Saturated Fat: 3 g, Trans fat: 0 g, Polyunsaturated Fat: 3 g, Monounsaturated Fat: 17 g, Cholesterol: 0 mg, Sodium: 240 mg, Total Carbohydrates: 54 g, Dietary Fiber: 8 g, Total Sugars: 15 g (including 3 g added sugar), Protein: 8 g

Fiesta Chopped Salad

MIND POINTS: 1 SERVING = 1 LG, 1 OV, 1 EVOO, 0.5 WG, 0.5 BN

I love a bright, colorful salad that holds up well to dressing and can be made ahead of time. This salad is great on its own as a side dish, or you can add your favorite protein to make it a main course.

Serves: 6
Prep time: 15 minutes

Salad:

- ¼ cup extra-virgin olive oil, or more as needed
- 3 corn tortillas, cut into ½-inch strips
- ¼ teaspoon salt
- 1 head romaine lettuce, cut into bite-size pieces
- 1 (15-ounce) can black beans, drained and rinsed
- 1 cup fresh, thawed frozen, or drained canned corn
- 1 cup halved cherry or grape tomatoes
- 1 cup chopped purple cabbage
- 1 bell pepper, seeded and cut into thin matchsticks

Dressing:

- ¼ cup extra-virgin olive oil
- 2 tablespoons apple cider vinegar
- 2 tablespoons tahini
- Grated zest and juice of 1 lime
- 1 teaspoon honey

Garnish:

- 1 avocado, peeled, pitted, and diced

3 tablespoons chopped fresh cilantro (optional)

2 tablespoons chopped jalapeños (optional)

¼ cup crumbled feta cheese (optional)

Heat the oil in a medium skillet over medium-high heat. Add 1 tortilla strip to test the oil. If the oil sizzles around the strip, it is ready. Add the strips one at a time, making sure not to crowd the pan. Cook for 30 seconds or until lightly golden, then flip and repeat. Add more oil if needed. Transfer to a paper towel–lined plate to drain. Top with a sprinkle of salt.

In a large bowl, combine the romaine, black beans, corn, tomatoes, cabbage, and bell pepper.

In a small bowl, whisk together all the dressing ingredients. Pour the dressing over the salad and toss lightly. Top with the avocado, crispy tortilla strips, cilantro, jalapeños, and feta, if desired.

Nutritional analysis per serving (serving size: 2 cups): Calories: 380, Total Fat: 26 g, Saturated Fat: 3.5 g, Trans fat: 0 g, Polyunsaturated Fat: 3.5 g, Monounsaturated Fat: 18 g, Cholesterol: 0 mg, Sodium: 220 mg, Total Carbohydrates: 35 g, Dietary Fiber: 10 g, Total Sugars: 5 g (including 1 g added sugar), Protein: 9 g

Roasted Kale Chips

MIND POINTS: 1 SERVING = 1 LG, 0.5 EVOO

Kale chips are a staple in our house. I would say we serve these at least once a week. My kids love to help pull the kale off the stems and rinse the leaves. These chips are super simple to make and a great way to get in your greens for the day.

Serves: 4
Prep time: 10 minutes
Cook time: 15 minutes

1 bunch curly kale

2 tablespoons extra-virgin olive oil

¼ teaspoon salt, plus more to taste

1 tablespoon nutritional yeast (optional)

Preheat the oven to 375°F. Line a rimmed baking sheet with aluminum foil.

Pull the kale leaves off the stems and tear into rough 1-inch pieces. Rinse the kale thoroughly, using your fingers to clean any dirt between the leaves. Dry the kale completely using a towel or salad spinner. This ensures it gets crisp and doesn't steam.

Spread out the kale on the prepared baking sheet. Drizzle with the oil and massage the kale so most of the leaves have a light coat of oil. Evenly space out the leaves, making sure not to crowd the sheet; use two baking sheets, if necessary. Sprinkle with the salt and nutritional yeast, if desired.

Bake for 12 to 15 minutes, until the kale is slightly golden at the edges and crispy. Sprinkle with a touch more salt, if desired.

Nutritional analysis per serving (serving size: ½ cup): Calories: 60, Total Fat: 6 g, Saturated Fat: 1 g, Trans fat: 0 g, Polyunsaturated Fat: 0.5 g, Monounsaturated Fat: 4.5 g, Cholesterol: 0 mg, Sodium: 180 mg, Total Carbohydrates: 2 g, Dietary Fiber: 1 g, Total Sugars: 0 g (including 0 g added sugar), Protein: 1 g

Creamy Spinach Dip

MIND POINTS: 1 SERVING = 0 MIND POINTS

This creamy dip is so good, you'd never know it doesn't have cheese or cream in it! Nutritional yeast gives it a cheesy taste, while the salsa and seasoning provide a little kick. This is a great, healthy alternative to traditional spinach dips, and it is just as satisfying. Although this recipe has no MIND points, it is a great substitute for traditional spinach dips that use cream cheese and butter. Serve warm with fresh veggies, pita bread, or tortilla chips.

Serves: 8
Prep time: 10 minutes
Cook time: 10 minutes

> 3 tablespoons avocado oil
>
> 4 garlic cloves, chopped
>
> ¼ cup all-purpose flour
>
> 1¾ cups milk of choice
>
> 5 tablespoons nutritional yeast
>
> ¼ teaspoon salt, plus more to taste
>
> ¼ teaspoon ground cumin
>
> ⅓ cup salsa
>
> ¼ cup chopped frozen spinach, thawed with excess water squeezed out, *or* 2 cups fresh spinach, finely chopped

Heat the oil in a medium saucepan over medium heat for about 1 minute. Add the garlic and cook for 30 to 60 seconds, stirring frequently so it doesn't burn.

Add the flour a tablespoon at a time and whisk over low heat. Continue whisking until a paste forms, about 1 minute after you add the last tablespoon of flour.

Slowly whisk in the milk until combined and creamy. Continue to whisk until the milk thickens, 2 to 3 minutes. It should coat the back of a spoon without dripping off right away. Whisk in the nutritional yeast, salt, and cumin until combined, about 1 minute.

Add the salsa and spinach. Stir to combine and remove from the heat. Season with more salt, if needed.

Nutritional analysis per serving (serving size: ¼ cup): Calories: 140, Total Fat: 8 g, Saturated Fat: 3 g, Trans fat: 0 g, Polyunsaturated Fat: 1 g, Monounsaturated Fat: 2 g, Cholesterol: 0 mg, Sodium: 300 mg, Total Carbohydrates: 12 g, Dietary Fiber: 2 g, Total Sugars: 3 g (including 2 g added sugar), Protein: 5 g

Spicy Black Bean Hummus

MIND POINTS: 1 SERVING = 1 EVOO, 1 BN

This spicy dip subs out chickpeas from traditional hummus for black beans. It gets eaten almost as quickly as I can make it. The recipe calls for pickled jalapeños to add some spice, but you can use fresh jalapeños if you prefer. If you have heat-sensitive eaters, you can forgo the jalapeños altogether, and this hummus is just as tasty. Serve with tortilla chips and fresh veggies.

Serves: 4
Prep time: 10 minutes

   1 (15-ounce) can black beans, drained and rinsed

   ¼ cup extra-virgin olive oil

   2 tablespoons tahini

   Juice of 1 lime

   ¼ cup loosely packed fresh cilantro, plus a few leaves for garnish

   1 garlic clove, peeled

   2 teaspoons ground coriander

   2 teaspoons ground cumin

   ½ teaspoon salt, or to taste

   ¼ cup sliced pickled jalapeños, plus a few slices for garnish

In a food processor, combine the black beans, oil, tahini, lime juice, cilantro, garlic, coriander, cumin, and salt. Blend until smooth (or slightly chunky if you prefer). Add the jalapeños and pulse until incorporated. Transfer to a bowl and garnish with cilantro and pickled jalapeños.

Nutritional analysis per serving (serving size: ¼ cup): Calories: 240, Total Fat: 18 g, Saturated Fat: 2.5 g, Trans fat: 0 g, Polyunsaturated Fat: 3 g, Monounsaturated Fat: 12 g, Cholesterol: 0 mg, Sodium: 420 mg, Total Carbohydrates: 15 g, Dietary Fiber: 6 g, Total Sugars: 0 g (including 0 g added sugar), Protein: 6 g

Olive Oil Popcorn

MIND POINTS: 1 SERVING= 1 EVOO, 1 WG

Popcorn and movie night was a favorite in my house growing up, and now it is with my kids, too. This popcorn is made with extra-virgin olive oil and seasoned with salt. It is delicious as is, or you can spruce it up by adding different toppings, such as a sprinkle of nutritional yeast, lemon pepper, cinnamon sugar, or chili powder, to name a few. Whatever you choose, it will not last long!

Serves: 4
Cook time: 5 minutes

   ¼ cup extra-virgin olive oil
   ½ cup popcorn kernels
   ¼ teaspoon salt

Heat the oil in a large, heavy-bottomed pot over medium heat. Add 2 popcorn kernels and cover until they pop—about 1 minute. Add the rest of the kernels and partially cover, leaving a little vent for air to escape. Lightly shimmy the pot and let the kernels start to warm in the oil. Once the kernels begin to pop, reduce the heat to medium-low and periodically give the pot a shimmy to prevent the kernels from burning.

You'll know the popcorn is done once 3 to 5 seconds go by without a pop. Take the pot off the heat immediately.

Transfer the popcorn to a large bowl and season with the salt, giving the bowl a little shake to evenly distribute the salt.

Nutritional analysis per serving (serving size: 3 cups): Calories: 150, Total Fat: 14 g, Saturated Fat: 2 g, Trans fat: 0 g, Polyunsaturated Fat: 2 g, Monounsaturated Fat: 10 g, Cholesterol: 0 mg, Sodium: 150 mg, Total Carbohydrates: 6 g, Dietary Fiber: 1 g, Total Sugars: 0 g (including 0 g added sugar), Protein: 1 g

CHAPTER 23

Sweets

Balsamic Berries

MIND POINTS: 1 SERVING = 1.5 BER

Our family had berries in the house year round. I love berries as they are, but marinating them makes them into more of a dessert. This dish is incredibly easy and sophisticated at the same time. It's vibrant in color and layered with flavor. Be sure to use a high-quality balsamic vinegar, one that has a mild tartness rather than strong acidity. When looking at the ingredient list, look for "grape must, tradizionale."

Serves: 6
Prep time: 5 minutes, plus 30 minutes to marinate

1 tablespoon sugar

1½ tablespoons balsamic vinegar

2 cups quartered strawberries

1 cup blueberries

1 cup raspberries

1 cup blackberries

1 to 2 tablespoons chopped fresh mint (optional)

In a small bowl, whisk together the sugar and balsamic vinegar.

Put the berries in a serving bowl. Drizzle the balsamic vinegar mixture over the berries and gently toss. Marinate in the fridge or on the countertop for at least 30 minutes. Garnish with the mint, if desired.

Nutritional analysis per serving (serving size: ¾ cup): Calories: 60, Total Fat: 0 g, Saturated Fat: 0 g, Trans fat: 0 g, Polyunsaturated Fat: 0 g, Monounsaturated Fat: 0 g, Cholesterol: 0 mg, Sodium: 0 mg, Total Carbohydrates: 15 g, Dietary Fiber: 4 g, Total Sugars: 10 g (including 2 g added sugar), Protein: 1 g

Olive Oil Banana Bread

MIND POINTS: 1 SERVING = 0.5 EVOO, 1 WG

There is nothing like the smell of freshly baked banana bread. In our house, we love to eat it with a pat of butter spread or peanut butter. The typical banana bread recipe calls for loads of sugar, butter, and white flour. This recipe switches out those ingredients for more brain-healthy foods, but keeps the flavor to perfection. This is the best way to use up those overripe bananas.

Makes: 1 loaf; 9 servings
Prep time: 10 minutes
Cook time: 55 minutes

⅓ cup extra-virgin olive oil

⅓ cup pure maple syrup

¼ cup sugar

2 eggs

1 cup mashed ripe bananas (2 to 3 bananas)

¼ cup milk of choice

1 teaspoon vanilla extract

1 teaspoon baking soda

½ teaspoon ground cinnamon

¼ teaspoon salt

1 cup spelt or oat flour

1 cup whole-wheat flour

½ cup chopped walnuts (optional)

¼ cup dark or semisweet chocolate chips (optional)

Preheat the oven to 325°F.

Lightly grease a 9-by-5-inch loaf pan with cooking spray or oil.

In a large bowl, whisk together the oil, maple syrup, and sugar. Add the eggs and beat well, then whisk in the mashed bananas and milk. Add the vanilla, baking soda, cinnamon, and salt and stir to combine.

Slowly fold in the flours until just combined—don't overmix. Fold in the chopped walnuts, if desired. Pour the batter into the prepared loaf pan. Sprinkle the chocolate chips on top, if desired.

Bake for 50 to 60 minutes, until a toothpick inserted into the center comes out clean. Let cool for at least 10 minutes.

Nutritional analysis per serving (serving size: 1-inch slice): Calories: 250, Total Fat: 10 g, Saturated Fat: 1.5 g, Trans fat: 0 g, Polyunsaturated Fat: 1 g, Monounsaturated Fat: 7 g, Cholesterol: 40 mg, Sodium: 220 mg, Total Carbohydrates: 36 g, Dietary Fiber: 3 g, Total Sugars: 15 g (including 13 g added sugar), Protein: 5 g

Pumpkin Pie Parfaits

MIND POINTS: 1 SERVING = 0.5 OV, 1 NUT

Calling all pumpkin pie lovers! These parfaits are so tasty and a much lighter version than a traditional pumpkin pie. I love that they can be prepared ahead of time and pulled out of the refrigerator just before serving, no need to bake. You can use any nut for your candied nut crunch layer. If you want to make this dish even lighter, you can use toasted nuts instead of candied. This recipe calls for coconut whipped cream, which is a tasty nondairy alternative that can be found in the frozen dessert section of most grocery stores.

Serves: 6
Prep time: 20 minutes
Cook time: 30 minutes

For the candied nuts:

- 3 cups raw almonds or nut of choice
- ⅓ cup pure maple syrup
- ½ teaspoon ground cinnamon
- ¼ teaspoon salt

For the pumpkin pie filling:

- ¼ cup cornstarch
- ⅓ cup brown sugar
- 2 cups milk of choice
- 1 (15-ounce) can pumpkin puree
- 2 tablespoons pure maple syrup
- ½ teaspoon vanilla extract
- 1½ teaspoons ground cinnamon
- ¼ teaspoon ground nutmeg
- ¼ teaspoon ground ginger
- ¼ teaspoon ground allspice

For the topping:

- ½ cup coconut whipped cream or whipped topping of choice
- 3 tablespoons cacao nibs

Preheat the oven to 325°F. Line a rimmed baking sheet with parchment paper.

To make the candied nuts, in a medium bowl, toss the almonds with the maple syrup, cinnamon, and salt until well coated. Spread the nuts out on the prepared baking sheet and roast for 10 minutes. Remove from the oven and stir the nuts with a wooden spoon. Return to the oven for another 15 minutes, taking the nuts out every 5 minutes or so to stir. Remove from the oven and let cool.

To make the filling, in a small saucepan set over low heat, stir the cornstarch and sugar together. Add 1 tablespoon milk at a time, whisking until a paste is formed, about 2 minutes. Add the remaining milk while whisking constantly to prevent clumping. Whisk for another 60 to 90 seconds, until no clumps are left.

Whisk in the pumpkin puree. Bring to a boil, then turn the heat down to a low simmer while continuing to whisk. Once the mixture has thickened, whisk in the maple syrup, vanilla, cinnamon, nutmeg, ginger, and allspice. Remove from the heat.

When the nuts have cooled, roughly chop them until they have a chunky crumb-like consistency.

In each of 6 serving bowls or small mason jars, layer about 2 tablespoons candied nuts, then about ¼ cup pumpkin mixture, followed by another 2 tablespoons nuts, then another layer of ¼ cup pumpkin mixture.

Top each serving with 1 tablespoon whipped topping and ½ tablespoon cacao nibs.

Nutritional analysis per serving (serving size: 1 parfait): Calories: 410, Total Fat: 23 g, Saturated Fat: 3.5 g, Trans fat: 0 g, Polyunsaturated Fat: 4.5 g, Monounsaturated Fat: 11 g, Cholesterol: 0 mg, Sodium: 140 mg, Total Carbohydrates: 47 g, Dietary Fiber: 9 g, Total Sugars: 25 g (including 20 g added sugar), Protein: 10 g

Protein Power Bites

MIND POINTS: 1 SERVING = 0.5 NUT

These little bites are perfect to have on hand for those with a sweet tooth or anyone who needs a good dose of carbohydrates and protein. You can make them without the protein powder and they are just as tasty. When shopping for protein powder, look for brands that are low in sugar (including replacement sugars such as sucralose). I like to use plant-based protein powder such as Vega brand. I enjoy vanilla-flavored but chocolate or unflavored works, too.

Makes: 12 bites
Prep time: 8 minutes

½ cup raw pecans

6 Medjool dates, pitted

⅓ cup natural peanut or other nut butter

1 scoop (about ⅓ cup) protein powder

1 tablespoon unsweetened cocoa powder

½ teaspoon ground cinnamon

¼ teaspoon salt

2 tablespoons milk of choice

2 tablespoons plus ⅓ cup hemp seeds

Put the pecans in a food processor and pulse until they have a sand-like texture. Transfer to a medium bowl.

Put the dates in the food processor and pulse until they are in very small pieces. (If they are very hard or dry, first soak them in hot water and drain.)

Add the peanut butter, protein powder, cocoa powder, cinnamon, salt, milk, and 2 tablespoons of the hemp seeds to the food processor with the dates. Pulse to mix.

Return the pecans to the food processor and pulse until well incorporated and almost smooth.

Scoop out a heaping tablespoon, roll into a ball, and place it on a baking sheet or plate. Continue until all the dough is rolled into balls. If your hands get sticky, rinse them and keep them a little wet.

Pour the remaining ⅓ cup hemp seeds onto a plate. Roll each ball in the hemp seeds until well coated. Store in an airtight container in the fridge for up to 5 days.

Nutritional analysis per serving (serving size: 2 bites): Calories: 310, Total Fat: 21 g, Saturated Fat: 2.5 g, Trans fat: 0 g, Polyunsaturated Fat: 7 g, Monounsaturated Fat: 4.5 g, Cholesterol: 0 mg, Sodium: 150 mg, Total Carbohydrates: 21 g, Dietary Fiber: 4 g, Total Sugars: 14 g (including 0 g added sugar), Protein: 13 g

Butterfinger Bites

MIND POINTS: 1 SERVING = 0.5 NUT

I love making these chocolaty treats for all kinds of occasions. They are a big hit and are better for you than a traditional chocolate bar. They are still a treat, though, so be sure to eat them in moderation! These store well in the freezer.

Makes: 22 bites
Prep time: 15 minutes, plus 30 minutes to chill

3 cups cornflakes

1 cup smooth natural peanut butter

⅓ cup pure maple syrup

1 teaspoon vanilla extract

1½ cups semisweet chocolate chips

In a food processor, pulse the cornflakes until they have a sand-like consistency. Transfer to a medium bowl and add the peanut butter, maple syrup, and vanilla. Mix until well incorporated.

Line a rimmed baking sheet with parchment paper. Using a spoon, scoop out a golf-ball-size amount of dough. Shape into a rectangle or oval and place it on the prepared baking sheet. Repeat with the remaining dough. Freeze until hardened, about 20 minutes.

While the dough is chilling, in a microwave-safe bowl, microwave the chocolate chips in 30-second intervals, stirring until the chocolate is just melted.

Using a fork, dip each peanut butter piece into the chocolate to coat, then place it back on the baking sheet. Using a spoon, drizzle the remaining chocolate over the pieces to make them a little more fancy (this part is optional!).

Chill in the refrigerator to harden the chocolate, about 10 minutes. Transfer to a container and refrigerate for up to 5 days, or keep frozen for a quick treat!

Nutritional analysis per serving (serving size: 1 bite): Calories: 160, Total Fat: 9 g, Saturated Fat: 3 g, Trans fat: 0 g, Polyunsaturated Fat: 2 g, Monounsaturated Fat: 4 g, Cholesterol: 5 mg, Sodium: 75 mg, Total Carbohydrates: 15 g, Dietary Fiber: 1 g, Total Sugars: 10 g (including 8 g added sugar), Protein: 4 g

Chickpea Skillet Bars

MIND POINTS: 1 SERVING = 0.5 NUT, 0.5 BN

These bars are a big hit with my kids. Since they are made with hearty chickpeas and oats, they are filling and energizing at the same time; they will not make you sluggish like regular cookies would. If you have a sweet tooth, these are great to have in the refrigerator for a satisfying, sweet bite.

Makes: 10 bars
Prep time: 10 minutes
Cook time: 25 minutes

¾ cup old-fashioned rolled oats

1 (15-ounce) can chickpeas, drained and rinsed

⅔ cup smooth natural peanut butter

½ cup pure maple syrup

⅓ cup milk of choice

1 tablespoon vanilla extract

½ teaspoon ground cinnamon

½ teaspoon salt

⅓ cup dark chocolate chips

Preheat the oven to 350°F.

Lightly grease an 8-inch cast-iron skillet or an 8-inch square baking pan with cooking spray or oil.

In a food processor, pulse the oats until they have a flour-like consistency. Add the chickpeas, peanut butter, maple syrup, milk, vanilla, cinnamon, and salt and blend until well combined and smooth. The batter should be thick and slightly sticky. Gently fold in ¼ cup of the chocolate chips (do not pulse).

Transfer the mixture to the prepared skillet or pan. Sprinkle the remaining chocolate chips on top.

Bake for 25 minutes, or until a toothpick inserted in the middle comes out clean. It's okay if it's slightly undercooked, as there is no egg, and it will continue to cook in the pan after it comes out of the oven.

Allow to cool. Cut into 10 bars and store in the refrigerator for up to 1 week.

Nutritional analysis per serving (serving size: 1 bar): Calories: 260, Total Fat: 12 g, Saturated Fat: 3 g, Trans fat: 0 g, Polyunsaturated Fat: 3 g, Monounsaturated Fat: 5 g, Cholesterol: 0 mg, Sodium: 230 mg, Total Carbohydrates: 28 g, Dietary Fiber: 4 g, Total Sugars: 15 g (including 13 g added sugar), Protein: 7 g

Chewy Oatmeal Chocolate Chip Cookies

MIND POINTS: 1 SERVING = 0.5 WG

In my opinion, there is nothing better than a delicious chocolate chip cookie. My family will tell you I started my culinary journey by baking batch after batch of different kinds of cookies, starting at around age 9. Chocolate chip cookies should be sweet and slightly chewy, and have that delicious, rich chocolate bite. Although this recipe has far less sugar and butter than a traditional chocolate chip cookie, you will hardly notice! I suggest using a "flax egg" in this recipe for two reasons. First, with the rise in food allergies it's a good idea to know how to modify a recipe to be more allergen-friendly; and second, it gives you an excuse to eat the cookie dough! If you want to use a regular egg, please do so; it works just as well.

Makes: 12 to 15 cookies
Prep time: 10 minutes
Cook time: 15 minutes

- 1 tablespoon flaxseeds
- 3 tablespoons water
- 1 cup oat, spelt, almond, or whole-wheat flour
- 1 cup old-fashioned rolled oats
- ½ teaspoon baking soda
- ½ teaspoon salt
- ¼ cup vegan butter or unsalted dairy butter
- ¼ cup almond or natural peanut butter
- ¼ cup brown sugar
- ¼ cup cane sugar
- ¼ cup pure maple syrup
- 1 teaspoon vanilla extract
- ⅓ cup dark or semisweet chocolate chips or chunks

Preheat the oven to 350°F. Line a rimmed baking sheet with parchment paper.

In a small bowl, whisk together the flaxseeds and water to make a flax "egg." Set aside.

In a large bowl, whisk together the flour, oats, baking soda, and salt.

In the bowl of an electric mixer, beat together the butter, almond butter, brown sugar, and cane sugar for about 2 minutes. Mix in the flax egg, maple syrup, and vanilla.

Gradually mix in the dry ingredients until just incorporated. Be sure not to overmix. Fold in the chocolate chips.

Shape the dough into 1-inch balls and place them on the prepared baking sheet, leaving about 2 inches between each ball.

Bake for 12 to 14 minutes, until just lightly golden around the edges. The cookies will come out soft and harden slightly as they cool.

Nutritional analysis per serving (serving size: 1 cookie): Calories: 200, Total Fat: 8 g, Saturated Fat: 4 g, Trans fat: 0 g, Polyunsaturated Fat: 2 g, Monounsaturated Fat: 3 g, Cholesterol: 9 mg, Sodium: 140 mg, Total Carbohydrates: 25 g, Dietary Fiber: 3 g, Total Sugars: 11 g (including 11 g added sugar), Protein: 5 g

CHAPTER 24

Sauces and Toppers

Arugula Pesto

MIND POINTS: 1 SERVING = 0.5 LG, 0.5 NUT

This pesto is so simple to make and tastes good on almost everything— sandwiches, pasta, chicken, or even with fresh veggies as a dip. You can substitute kale for the arugula and it will taste just as good.

Serves: 6
Prep time: 7 minutes

> 2½ cups arugula
>
> ⅓ cup unsalted raw walnuts
>
> ½ cup extra-virgin olive oil
>
> Grated zest and juice of 1 lime or lemon
>
> ½ teaspoon salt

Combine all the ingredients in a food processor or blender and blend until smooth. Store in an airtight container in the refrigerator for up to 5 days.

Nutritional analysis per serving (serving size: ¼ cup): Calories: 210, Total Fat: 22 g, Saturated Fat: 3 g, Trans fat: 0 g, Polyunsaturated Fat: 4.5 g, Monounsaturated Fat: 15 g, Cholesterol: 0 mg, Sodium: 200 mg, Total Carbohydrates: 2 g, Dietary Fiber: 1 g, Total Sugars: 0 g (including 0 g added sugar), Protein: 1 g

Garlicky Yogurt Sauce

MIND POINTS: 1 SERVING = 0.5 OV

This sauce adds a creamy texture and bright, bold flavors to your favorite dishes. It is a good substitute for higher-calorie dressings such as ranch and Caesar. This recipe has cucumbers, but it is just as good without them!

Makes: 1½ cups
Prep time: 5 minutes

1 cup 2% plain Greek yogurt

¼ cup chopped fresh parsley

1 garlic clove, chopped

Juice of 1 lemon

2 mini cucumbers, finely chopped

¼ teaspoon salt

¼ teaspoon black pepper

In a medium bowl, combine all the ingredients and mix well. Cover and store in the refrigerator for up to 5 days.

Nutritional analysis per serving (serving size: 3 tablespoons): Calories: 35, Total Fat: 1 g, Saturated Fat: 0.5 g, Trans fat: 0 g, Polyunsaturated Fat: 0 g, Monounsaturated Fat: 0 g, Cholesterol: 0 mg, Sodium: 0 mg, Total Carbohydrates: 3 g, Dietary Fiber: 0 g, Total Sugars: 1 g (including 0 g added sugar), Protein: 4 g

Creamy Tahini Sauce

MIND POINTS: 1 SERVING = 1 NUT

Tahini is a smooth, creamy sesame seed butter with a pourable consistency. This sauce is so incredibly simple, and it goes well with many dishes. It can be used as a substitute for sour cream, cheese sauces, and ranch dip; it's a great way to get a more decadent sauce without using animal fats such as butter or cream.

Makes: 2 cups
Prep time: 3 minutes

- 2 garlic cloves, minced
- ¼ teaspoon salt
- ¼ cup lemon juice
- 1 cup tahini
- 1 teaspoon ground cumin
- ¾ cup cold water

In a medium bowl, combine the garlic, salt, and lemon juice and let sit for 1 minute. Whisk in the tahini and cumin until just incorporated. Whisk in the cold water, ¼ cup at a time, until the sauce is smooth and creamy. Cover and store in the refrigerator for up to 1 week.

Nutritional analysis per serving (serving size: 2 tablespoons): Calories: 180, Total Fat: 16 g, Saturated Fat: 2 g, Trans fat: 0 g, Polyunsaturated Fat: 7 g, Monounsaturated Fat: 6 g, Cholesterol: 0 mg, Sodium: 110 mg, Total Carbohydrates: 7 g, Dietary Fiber: 3 g, Total Sugars: 0 g (including 0 g added sugar), Protein: 5 g

Soy-Sriracha Stir-Fry Sauce

MIND POINTS: 1 SERVING = 0.5 EVOO

This is a great all-purpose sauce to use over vegetables, noodles, grains, and proteins such as fish or chicken.

Makes: ¾ cup
Prep time: 5 minutes

- ¼ cup low-sodium soy sauce
- ¼ cup extra-virgin olive oil
- 2 tablespoons sriracha
- 2 tablespoons honey
- ½ teaspoon chili paste, or to taste

In a medium bowl, whisk together all the ingredients. Cover and refrigerate in an airtight container for up to 1 week.

Nutritional analysis per serving (serving size: 2 tablespoons): Calories: 160, Total Fat: 14 g, Saturated Fat: 2 g, Trans fat: 0 g, Polyunsaturated Fat: 1.5 g, Monounsaturated Fat: 11 g, Cholesterol: 0 mg, Sodium: 550 mg, Total Carbohydrates: 8 g, Dietary Fiber: 0 g, Total Sugars: 6 g (including 5 g added sugar), Protein: 1 g

Balsamic Reduction

MIND POINTS: 1 SERVING = 0 MIND POINTS

Balsamic reduction is a delicious way to add depth and flavor to a dish. You can drizzle it over vegetables, fruit, fish, or grains—it is so versatile. The highest-quality balsamic vinegar comes from Modena and Reggio Emilia in Italy. The vinegar should reduce to a quarter of its volume, leaving a glossy sauce. You want it to be pourable—a similar consistency to warm honey. This reduction has no MIND points, but you can use it in place of sugary dressings or drizzle it over dessert instead of caramel or chocolate sauce. You can make it a little sweeter by adding 1 tablespoon honey, which will make it more of a glaze, or flavor it with a small sprig of rosemary.

Makes: ¼ cup
Cook time: 15 minutes

1 cup balsamic vinegar

In a small saucepan, bring the vinegar to a simmer over low heat. Be careful not to bring it to a high simmer as it could burn easily. Also be prepared for a strong vinegar smell in your kitchen!

Whisk the vinegar frequently for 8 to 12 minutes, until it thickens and reduces by more than half. When it drips slowly off the back of a spoon, remove the pan from the heat. The sauce will continue to thicken as it cools.

When slightly cooled, carefully pour it into a clean glass jar with a lid and store it in the pantry (no need to refrigerate). When ready to serve, if the reduction is too thick, you can add a tablespoon or two of water over low heat to thin it out.

Nutritional analysis per serving (serving size: ¼ cup): Calories: 20, Total Fat: 0 g, Saturated Fat: 0 g, Trans fat: 0 g, Polyunsaturated Fat: 0 g, Monounsaturated Fat: 0 g, Cholesterol: 0 mg, Sodium: 0 mg, Total Carbohydrates: 8 g, Dietary Fiber: 0 g, Total Sugars: 8 g (including 0 g added sugar), Protein: 0 g

Goes with Everything Dressing

MIND POINTS: 1 SERVING = 1.5 EVOO

This is my go-to dressing for my everyday salads, for grains, for drizzling over cooked chicken and fish, and more. You can customize the flavor by adding Dijon mustard, tahini, mayonnaise, Greek yogurt, peanut butter, soy sauce, fresh herbs, shallots, or garlic. You can also change up the acid by using lemon or lime juice, balsamic vinegar, red wine vinegar—almost any variation will work. Just keep in mind that a typical salad dressing has a ratio of three parts oil to one part vinegar.

Makes: ¼ cup
Prep time: 2 minutes

> 3 tablespoons extra-virgin olive oil
>
> 1 tablespoon apple cider vinegar
>
> 2 teaspoons honey
>
> Pinch salt

In a small bowl, whisk together all the ingredients. (Alternatively, you can combine the ingredients in a small jar, cover, and shake until emulsified.) Store in the refrigerator for up to 2 weeks.

Nutritional analysis per serving (serving size: 2 tablespoons): Calories: 210, Total Fat: 21 g, Saturated Fat: 3 g, Trans fat: 0 g, Polyunsaturated Fat: 2 g, Monounsaturated Fat: 16 g, Cholesterol: 0 mg, Sodium: 150 mg, Total Carbohydrates: 6 g, Dietary Fiber: 0 g, Total Sugars: 5 g (including 5 g added sugar), Protein: 0 g

Regal Lemon-Shallot Dressing

MIND POINTS: 1 SERVING = 1 EVOO

This delicious dressing pairs nicely with most salads. It has a neutral balance of flavors that enhances chicken, roasted vegetables, or cooked grains.

Makes: 1 cup
Prep time: 4 minutes

½ cup lemon juice

¼ cup extra-virgin olive oil

2 tablespoons minced shallot

1 tablespoon minced fresh parsley *or* 1 teaspoon dried

1 tablespoon Dijon mustard

1½ teaspoons honey

In a medium bowl, whisk together all the ingredients until incorporated. Cover and store in the refrigerator for up to 5 days.

Nutritional analysis per serving (serving size: ¼ cup): Calories: 280, Total Fat: 27 g, Saturated Fat: 4 g, Trans fat: 0 g, Polyunsaturated Fat: 3 g, Monounsaturated Fat: 20 g, Cholesterol: 0 mg, Sodium: 89 mg, Total Carbohydrates: 11 g, Dietary Fiber: 1 g, Total Sugars: 6 g (including 1 g added sugar), Protein: 1 g

Pickled Red Onions

MIND POINTS: 1 SERVING = 0.5 OV

This quick pickled red onion recipe is so simple yet so elegant. You can customize it by adding your favorite flavors, like herbs, garlic, peppercorns, or vegetables that you love. If you have a mandoline slicer, this is a great time to use it! The thinner the onion slices, the better. I like to keep a jar of these in the refrigerator to add to sandwiches, salads, tacos, and dips.

Makes: 2 cups
Prep time: 5 minutes, plus 30 minutes to marinate
Cook time: 5 minutes

¾ cup apple cider vinegar

¼ cup water

1 tablespoon sugar

1 teaspoon salt

1 large red onion, very thinly sliced

In a medium saucepan, whisk together the vinegar, water, sugar, and salt. Bring to a simmer over medium heat and simmer for 2 minutes. Remove from the heat.

Put the onion slices in a small mason jar or other container. Carefully pour the hot brine over the onions. Gently push the onions down so they are mostly submerged. Cover and marinate at room temperature for 30 minutes. Store in the refrigerator for up to 2 weeks.

Nutritional analysis per serving (serving size: ¼ cup): Calories: 10, Total Fat: 0 g, Saturated Fat: 0 g, Trans fat: 0 g, Polyunsaturated Fat: 0 g, Monounsaturated Fat: 0 g, Cholesterol: 0 mg, Sodium: 75 mg, Total Carbohydrates: 3 g, Dietary Fiber: 0 g, Total Sugars: 2 g (including 1 g added sugar), Protein: 0 g

Toasted Nuts

MIND POINTS: 1 SERVING = 1 NUT

Toasting nuts draws the oils to the surface, intensifying the flavor and color while adding a little more crunch. Sprinkling toasted nuts on a dish can enhance the flavor and texture. I like to use toasted nuts in place of full-fat cheeses or meats on salads, sautéed veggies, and pastas. My go-to method is on the stovetop as it requires the fewest number of steps. You can also toast nuts in the oven to ensure even cooking. This recipe is for pine nuts, but you can toast any nut or seed using this method, although the timing may need to be adjusted.

Makes: ¼ cup
Cook time: 5 minutes

¼ cup pine nuts

Heat a small skillet over medium-low heat. When hot, add the pine nuts and shake the pan, or use a wooden spoon to swirl the nuts every 30 to 60 seconds. You will start to see the nuts turn a golden brown. Continue to swirl every 30 to 60 seconds until the nuts are consistently golden brown, 5 to 7 minutes total. If the nuts start to turn dark, transfer to a plate right away. Let cool, then store in an airtight container in the pantry or refrigerator for up to 2 weeks.

Nutritional analysis per serving (serving size: ¼ cup): Calories: 115, Total Fat: 11 g, Saturated Fat: 1 g, Trans fat: 0 g, Polyunsaturated Fat: 6 g, Monounsaturated Fat: 3 g, Cholesterol: 0 mg, Sodium: 0 mg, Total Carbohydrates: 2 g, Dietary Fiber: 1 g, Total Sugars: 0 g (including 0 g added sugar), Protein: 2 g

Acknowledgments

By Laura Morris and Jennifer Ventrelle

This book is a collaboration of so many brilliant individuals. First and foremost, thank you to Dr. Christy Tangney, who has been a mentor to both of us in so many ways over the years. Your knowledge on nutrition is unsurpassed. Thank you for sharing your time and expertise. Thank you to Leah Johnston for your help on nutritional analysis throughout the book. To the many people who worked on the MIND diet intervention trial, in particular Dr. Lisa Barnes, Dr. Frank Sacks, Chiquia Hollings, Dr. Neelum Aggarwal, Dr. Puja Agarwal, Dr. Thomas Holland, Dr. Xiaoran Liu, and Dr. Klodian Dhana, we thank you for your support and contributions on this important work. To our food photographers, Martina Drea and Briana Reamer, thank you for adding beautiful photos, and thanks to Sean Lara for the superb book cover. Thank you to our agents at Park and Fine, including Celeste Fine, John Maas, and Mia Vitale, for your efforts on behalf of this book. We are also thankful for the writer's touch provided by Jennifer Kasius. We must also give a huge thank-you to our very patient editor, Tracy Behar, as we worked through the creation of this book. Most importantly, thank you to the late Dr. Martha Clare Morris for inspiring us to show up, work hard, and share our passions.

By Laura Morris

I must start by thanking my writing partner, Jennifer Ventrelle. Creating this book was certainly a challenge, and your commitment to making it the very best shows your dedication to your work, the scientific field, and your passion for helping people. Thank you for all that you have done. Thank you to my sister, Clare Ramirez, and my brother, Patrick Morris, for entrusting me to tell the story of our mother's work. Our losses have been great, but our foundation of love and strength has been greater. I admire you both so much. To Rachel Morris, my dear sister-in-law, who has been one of my biggest supporters, cheerleaders, and confidants, thank you for putting up with this crazy family with love and patience.

This book would not have happened without the unwavering support of my husband, Dr. Darcy Marr. You are the most steadfast, protective, and supportive partner. Thank you for standing by my side as I maneuvered this emotional ride and everything in between. To my children, Nolan, Kelly, and Lylah, I wrote this book so one day you will have an idea of how amazing your grandmother was, and the impact she had on the world of nutrition and dementia. She loved you so much, and you and your cousins were by far her greatest joy in her final years. To my father, James Morris, who lived like it was heaven on earth, thank you for teaching me that joy is our greatest companion in life. Lastly, to my mother, Dr. Martha Clare Morris, who lived life to the absolute fullest, leaving no rock unturned. Being under your wing was my greatest privilege and honor. I promised you I would have an amazing life and give it all that I've got. Thank you for showing me the way.

By Jennifer Ventrelle

I will be forever grateful to Dr. Martha Clare Morris for bringing me into the world of nutrition and brain health and giving me the opportunity to be at the forefront of this exciting research. Thank you, MCM, for pouring your heart into this work and allowing me to learn from your wisdom and be guided by your grace. To another inspirationally brilliant nutritionist and professor, Dr. Christy Tangney: as my thesis advisor in graduate school and first mentor, Christy will always be someone to cherish—as a scientist, mentor, friend, and overall loving and kind human being. Thank you, Dr. T, for all that makes you who you are and for inspiring young women to achieve nothing short of greatness.

Reflecting on the expansion of my career beyond nutrition into physical activity, I again find myself feeling grateful for the Morris family. My early memories of Laura include her showing participants how easy it is to be active with nothing more than a sturdy chair, your own body weight, and a good attitude. Thank you, Laura, for being my teacher so many years ago and for trusting me today to write about my role as a tiny droplet in the huge wave that your mother has made in the field of diet and dementia.

I'd like to thank some very important women for their work on the MIND diet trial. First, Leah Johnston. Aside from her brilliance as a dietitian, all things process, organization, aesthetic, team building, technology, humor, and well...*fun* led back to Leah. Thank you, Leah, for reminding us all that life is meant to be joyful. Alongside Leah were the best team of nutrition case managers, who not only coached our participants with scientific rigor and enthusiasm but also endured all the literature reviews, curriculum revisions, unanswered help desk tickets, eight weeks of "optional" mindfulness meditation sessions, and one viral Instagram video. Thank you, Kristie Miller, Rachel Cohen, Briana Reamer, Megan Claysen, Beth Lukaszewicz, Sarah Ehlers, and Sarah Graef: you'll always be "the OGs." You truly made Dr. Morris's life work come to fruition.

To the MIND diet trial participants, from "Diet A" to "Diet B," thank you for the sacrifices made in the name of science — a combined total of 50 hours of fasting, 70 vials of blood, 60 cognitive exams, 41 hours on the phone with a dietitian, and 3+ years of your precious time. Each and every one of you has played a role in helping us explore the problem of Alzheimer's disease and be a part of its solution.

And finally, to my foundation. To my mother, Adrienne Ventrelle, thank you for teaching me that food is a gift that should be prepared with intention and shared with love. As a single mother who raised three children and still managed to prepare home-cooked meals every night, your endless devotion and unwavering support taught me unconditional love. To my partner, Jason Pullman, your patience and kind heart are truly ethereal. Thank you for loving me through all the moments—inspirational, creative, irritable, and catastrophic alike. The hours spent writing with you and Lorenzo by my side through indoor summer weekends, shortened vacations, and canceled dinner plans were the fuel that kept me believing in myself and our future.

Notes

Introduction: The Dinner Table

1. Morris MC, Tangney CC, Wang Y, Sacks FM, Bennett DA, Aggarwal NT. MIND diet associated with reduced incidence of Alzheimer's disease. *Alzheimers Dement.* 2015;11(9):1007–1014
2. The MIND Diet: 2023 Guide for Alzheimer's & Brain Health | U.S. News Best Diets. *US News & World Report.* Accessed May 21, 2023. https://health.usnews.com/best-diet/mind-diet
3. Morris DMC. *Diet for the MIND: The Latest Science on What to Eat to Prevent Alzheimer's and Cognitive Decline.* New York: Little, Brown Spark; 2017

Chapter 1: The Problem of Alzheimer's Disease — and Its Solution?

1. 2022 Alzheimer's disease facts and figures. First published: 14 March 2022. *Alzheimers Dement.* 2022;18(4):700–789. https://doi.org/10.1002/alz.12638.
2. 2022 Alzheimer's disease facts and figures. *Alzheimers Dement.* 2022;18(4):700–789. doi:10.1002/alz.12638

Chapter 2: The Research on Nutrients for the Brain

1. Bienias JL, Beckett LA, Bennett DA, Wilson RS, Evans DA. Design of the Chicago Health and Aging Project (CHAP). *J Alzheimers Dis.* 2003;5(5):349-355. doi:10.3233/JAD-2003-5501
2. Morris MC. The role of nutrition in Alzheimer's disease: epidemiological evidence. *Eur J Neurol.* 2009;16:1-7. doi:10.1111/j.1468-1331.2009.02735.x
3. Bennett DA, Schneider JA, Buchman AS, Barnes LL, Boyle PA, Wilson RS. Overview and findings from the Rush Memory and Aging Project. *Curr Alzheimer Res.* 2012;9(6):646-663. doi:10.2174/156720512801322663
4. Morris MC, Schneider JA, Li H, et al. Brain tocopherols related to Alzheimer's disease neuropathology in humans. *Alzheimers Dement.* 2015;11(1):32-39. doi:10.1016/j.jalz.2013.12.015

5. Boccardi V, Baroni M, Mangialasche F, Mecocci P. Vitamin E family: Role in the pathogenesis and treatment of Alzheimer's disease. *Alzheimers Dement Transl Res Clin Interv.* 2016;2(3):182-191. doi:10.1016/j.trci.2016.08.002

6. Morris MC, Brockman J, Schneider JA, et al. Association of seafood consumption, brain mercury level, and APOE ε4 status with brain neuropathology in older adults. *JAMA.* 2016;315(5):489. doi:10.1001/jama.2016.19451;
   van de Rest O, Wang Y, Barnes LL, Tangney C, Bennett DA, Morris MC. APOE ε4 and the associations of seafood and long-chain omega-3 fatty acids with cognitive decline. *Neurology.* 2016;86(22):2063-2070. doi:10.1212/WNL.0000000000002719

7. Morris MC, Schneider JA, Tangney CC. Thoughts on B-vitamins and dementia. *J Alzheimers Dis JAD.* 2006;9(4):429-433. doi:10.3233/jad-2006-9409

8. Wang Z, Zhu W, Xing Y, Jia J, Tang Y. B vitamins and prevention of cognitive decline and incident dementia: a systematic review and meta-analysis. *Nutr Rev.* 2022;80(4):931-949. doi:10.1093/nutrit/nuab057

9. Morris MC. Diet and Alzheimer's disease: what the evidence shows. *Medscape Gen Med.* 2004;6(1):48;
   Ruan Y, Tang J, Guo X, Li K, Li D. Dietary fat intake and risk of Alzheimer's disease and dementia: a meta-analysis of cohort studies. *Curr Alzheimer Res.* 2018;15(9):869-876. doi:10.2174/1567205015666180427142350

10. Yuan C, Chen H, Wang Y, Schneider JA, Willett WC, Morris MC. Dietary carotenoids related to risk of incident Alzheimer dementia (AD) and brain AD neuropathology: a community-based cohort of older adults. *Am J Clin Nutr.* 2021;113(1):200-208. doi:10.1093/ajcn/nqaa303

11. Shishtar E, Rogers GT, Blumberg JB, Au R, Jacques PF. Long-term dietary flavonoid intake and risk of Alzheimer disease and related dementias in the Framingham Offspring Cohort. *Am J Clin Nutr.* 2020;112(2):343-353. doi:10.1093/ajcn/nqaa079

12. National Institutes of Health, Office of Dietary Supplements. Vitamin D. Accessed May 1, 2023. ods.od.nih.gov/factsheets/VitaminD-HealthProfessional/

13. Shea MK, Barger K, Dawson-Hughes B, et al. Brain vitamin D forms, cognitive decline, and neuropathology in community-dwelling older adults. *Alzheimers Dement J Alzheimers Assoc.* Published online December 7, 2022. doi:10.1002/alz.12836

Chapter 3: The MIND Diet and Its Evidence for Protection against Neurodegenerative Diseases

1. Morris MC, Tangney CC, Wang Y, et al. MIND diet slows cognitive decline with aging. *Alzheimers Dement.* 2015;11(9):1015-1022. doi:10.1016/j.jalz.2015.04.011

2. Morris MC, Tangney CC, Wang Y, Sacks FM, Bennett DA, Aggarwal NT. MIND diet associated with reduced incidence of Alzheimer's disease. *Alzheimers Dement.* 2015;11(9):1007-1014. doi:10.1016/j.jalz.2014.11.009

3. Liu X, Morris MC, Dhana K, et al. Mediterranean-DASH Intervention for Neurodegenerative Delay (MIND) study: rationale, design and baseline characteristics of a randomized control trial of the MIND diet on cognitive decline. *Contemp Clin Trials.* 2021;102:106270. doi:10.1016/j.cct.2021.106270

Chapter 5: The Loss of a Great Leader

1. Barnes LL, Dhana K, Liu X, et al. (2023). Trial of the MIND diet for prevention of cognitive decline in older persons. *New Engl J Med*. 2023. Advance online publication. doi:10.1056/NEJMoa2302368
2. Morris MC, Tangney CC, Wang Y, Sacks FM, Bennett DA, Aggarwal NT. MIND diet associated with reduced incidence of Alzheimer's disease. *Alzheimers Dement*. 2015;11(9):1007-1014. doi:10.1016/j.jalz.2014.11.009
3. Morris MC, Tangney CC, Wang Y, et al. MIND diet slows cognitive decline with aging. *Alzheimers Dement*. 2015;11(9):1015-1022. doi:10.1016/j.jalz.2015.04.011

Chapter 6: Exciting New Research on the MIND Diet

1. Livingston G, Huntley J, Sommerlad A, et al. Dementia prevention, intervention, and care: 2020 report of the Lancet Commission. *Lancet Lond Engl*. 2020;396(10248):413-446. doi:10.1016/S0140-6736(20)30367-6
2. Ngandu T, Lehtisalo J, Solomon A, et al. A 2 year multidomain intervention of diet, exercise, cognitive training, and vascular risk monitoring versus control to prevent cognitive decline in at-risk elderly people (FINGER): a randomised controlled trial. *Lancet Lond Engl*. 2015;385(9984):2255-2263. doi:10.1016/S0140-6736(15)60461-5
3. University of Eastern Finland. World-Wide FINGERS: the first global initiative for prevention of dementia and Alzheimer's disease. July 8, 2020. uef.fi/en/article/world-wide-fingers-the-first-global-initiative-for-prevention-of-dementia-and-alzheimers-disease
4. Cherian L, Wang Y, Fakuda K, Leurgans S, Aggarwal N, Morris M. Mediterranean-Dash Intervention for Neurodegenerative Delay (MIND) diet slows cognitive decline after stroke. *J Prev Alzheimers Dis*. 2019;6(4):267-273. doi:10.14283/jpad.2019.28
5. Morris MC, Tangney CC, Wang Y, Barnes LL, Bennett D, Aggarwal N. O2-02-04: Mind diet score more predictive than Dash or Mediterranean diet scores. *Alzheimers Dement*. 2014;10(4S_Part_2):P166-P166. doi:10.1016/j.jalz.2014.04.164
6. Mancini JG, Filion KB, Atallah R, Eisenberg MJ. Systematic review of the Mediterranean diet for long-term weight loss. *Am J Med*. 2016;129(4):407-415. e4. doi:10.1016/j.amjmed.2015.11.028;
Soltani S, Shirani F, Chitsazi MJ, Salehi-Abargouei A. The effect of dietary approaches to stop hypertension (DASH) diet on weight and body composition in adults: a systematic review and meta-analysis of randomized controlled clinical trials. 2016;17(5):442-454. doi:10.1111/obr.12391
7. US Department of Veterans Affairs. Management of adult overweight and obesity. Accessed January 30, 2023. healthquality.va.gov/guidelines/CD/obesity/
8. Holland TM, Agarwal P, Wang Y, et al. Association of dietary intake of flavonols with changes in global cognition and several cognitive abilities. *Neurology*. 2023;100(7):e694-e702. doi:10.1212/WNL.0000000000201541

9. Agarwal P, Leurgans SE, Agrawal S, et al. Association of Mediterranean-DASH intervention for neurodegenerative delay and Mediterranean diets with Alzheimer disease pathology. *Neurology.* Published online March 8, 2023:10 .1212/WNL.0000000000207176. doi:10.1212/WNL.0000000000207176

10. Agarwal P, Holland TM, James BD, et al. Pelargonidin and berry intake association with Alzheimer's disease neuropathology: a community-based study. *J Alzheimers Dis JAD.* 2022;88(2):653-661. doi:10.3233/JAD-215600

11. The MIND Diet: 2023 Guide for Alzheimer's & Brain Health. *US News & World Report.* Accessed January 10, 2023. health.usnews.com/best-diet/mind-diet

Chapter 7: NeverMIND the Diet

1. Pagoto SL, Appelhans BM. A call for an end to the diet debates. *JAMA.* 2013;310(7):687-688. doi:10.1001/jama.2013.8601;
Ge L, Sadeghirad B, Ball GDC, et al. Comparison of dietary macronutrient patterns of 14 popular named dietary programmes for weight and cardiovascular risk factor reduction in adults: systematic review and network meta-analysis of randomised trials. *BMJ.* 2020;369:m696. doi:10.1136/bmj.m696

2. Morris MC, Tangney CC, Wang Y, Sacks FM, Bennett DA, Aggarwal NT. MIND diet associated with reduced incidence of Alzheimer's disease. *Alzheimers Dement.* 2015;11(9):1007-1014. doi:10.1016/j.jalz.2014.11.009

3. Barnes LL, Dhana K, Liu X, et al. (2023). Trial of the MIND diet for prevention of cognitive decline in older persons. *New Engl J Med.* 2023. Advance online publication. doi:10.1056/NEJMoa2302368

Chapter 8: Vegetables (Plural) and Fruit (Singular)

1. Morris MC, Wang Y, Barnes LL, Bennett DA, Dawson-Hughes B, Booth SL. Nutrients and bioactives in green leafy vegetables and cognitive decline: Prospective study. *Neurology.* 2018;90(3):e214-e222. doi:10.1212/WNL.0000000000004815

2. Agarwal P, Leurgans SE, Agrawal S, et al. Association of Mediterranean-DASH intervention for neurodegenerative delay and Mediterranean diets with Alzheimer disease pathology. *Neurology.* Published online March 8, 2023:10.1212 /WNL.0000000000207176. doi:10.1212/WNL.0000000000207176

3. Nooyens ACJ, Bueno-de-Mesquita HB, van Boxtel MPJ, van Gelder BM, Verhagen H, Verschuren WMM. Fruit and vegetable intake and cognitive decline in middle-aged men and women: the Doetinchem Cohort Study. *Br J Nutr.* 2011;106(5):752-761. doi:10.1017/S0007114511001024

4. Devore EE, Kang JH, Breteler MMB, Grodstein F. Dietary intakes of berries and flavonoids in relation to cognitive decline. *Ann Neurol.* 2012;72(1):135-143. doi:10.1002/ana.23594

5. Samieri C, Sun Q, Townsend MK, Rimm EB, Grodstein F. Dietary flavonoid intake at midlife and healthy aging in women. *Am J Clin Nutr.* 2014;100(6):1489-1497. doi:10.3945/ajcn.114.085605

6. Agarwal P, Holland TM, James BD, et al. Pelargonidin and berry intake association with Alzheimer's disease neuropathology: a community-based study. *J Alzheimers Dis JAD*. 2022;88(2):653-661. doi:10.3233/JAD-215600
7. Bennett DA, Schneider JA, Buchman AS, Barnes LL, Boyle PA, Wilson SR. Overview and Findings from the Rush Memory and Aging Project. *Curr Alzheimer Res*. 2012;9(6):646-663. doi:10.2174/156720512801322663

Chapter 9: Unsaturated Fats: Extra-Virgin Olive Oil, Nuts, and Nut Butters

1. American Heart Association. Dietary Fats. Accessed April 27, 2022. heart.org/en/healthy-living/healthy-eating/eat-smart/fats/dietary-fats
2. Ambra R, Lucchetti S, Pastore G. A review of the effects of olive oil-cooking on phenolic compounds. *Molecules*. 2022;27(3):661. doi:10.3390/molecules27030661
3. De Alzaa F, Guillaume C, Ravetti L. Evaluation of chemical and physical changes in different commercial oils during heating. *Acta Sci Nutr Health*. 2018;2(6):2-11.
4. Martínez-Lapiscina EH, Clavero P, Toledo E, et al. Mediterranean diet improves cognition: the PREDIMED-NAVARRA randomised trial. *J Neurol Neurosurg Psychiatry*. 2013;84(12):1318-1325. doi:10.1136/jnnp-2012-304792;
Valls-Pedret C, Sala-Vila A, Serra-Mir M, et al. Mediterranean diet and age-related cognitive decline: a randomized clinical trial. *JAMA Intern Med*. 2015;175(7):1094-1103. doi:10.1001/jamainternmed.2015.1668

Chapter 10: Proteins: Fish and Poultry

1. Li Y, Li S, Wang W, Zhang D. Association between dietary protein intake and cognitive function in adults aged 60 years and older. *J Nutr Health Aging*. 2020;24(2):223-229. doi:10.1007/s12603-020-1317-4
2. Yeh TS, Yuan C, Ascherio A, Rosner BA, Blacker D, Willett WC. Long-term dietary protein intake and subjective cognitive decline in US men and women. *Am J Clin Nutr*. 2022;115(1):199-210. doi:10.1093/ajcn/nqab236
3. Li F, Liu X, Zhang D. Fish consumption and risk of depression: a meta-analysis. *J Epidemiol Community Health*. 2016;70(3):299-304. doi:10.1136/jech-2015-206278
4. Morris MC, Tangney CC, Wang Y, et al. MIND diet slows cognitive decline with aging. *Alzheimers Dement*. 2015;11(9):1015-1022. doi:10.1016/j.jalz.2015.04.011
5. Dennett C. Seafood: fishing for answers. *Today's Dietitian*. Accessed May 21, 2023. todaysdietitian.com/newarchives/0317p16.shtml
6. Del Moral AM, Fortique F. Omega-3 fatty acids and cognitive decline: a systematic review. *Nutr Hosp*. Published online 2019. doi:10.20960/nh.02496
7. AARP. Summer 2021 update to AARP's supplement survey. doi:10.26419/pia.00094.001
8. Morris MC, Evans DA, Bienias JL, et al. Dietary niacin and the risk of incident Alzheimer's disease and of cognitive decline. *J Neurol Neurosurg Psychiatry*. 2004;75(8):1093-1099. doi:10.1136/jnnp.2003.025858

9. Leidy HJ, Clifton PM, Astrup A, et al. The role of protein in weight loss and maintenance. *Am J Clin Nutr.* 2015;101(6):1320S-1329S. doi:10.3945/ajcn.114.084038

10. Hansen TT, Astrup A, Sjödin A. Are dietary proteins the key to successful body weight management? A systematic review and meta-analysis of studies assessing body weight outcomes after interventions with increased dietary protein. *Nutrients.* 2021;13(9):3193. doi:10.3390/nu13093193

11. Kim JE, O'Connor LE, Sands LP, Slebodnik MB, Campbell WW. Effects of dietary protein intake on body composition changes after weight loss in older adults: a systematic review and meta-analysis. *Nutr Rev.* 2016;74(3):210-224. doi:10.1093/nutrit/nuv065

Chapter 11: Carbohydrates: Whole Grains, Beans, and Legumes

1. Muth AK, Park SQ. The impact of dietary macronutrient intake on cognitive function and the brain. *Clin Nutr Edinb Scotl.* 2021;40(6):3999-4010. doi:10.1016/j.clnu.2021.04.043

2. Wengreen H, Munger RG, Cutler A, et al. Prospective study of Dietary Approaches to Stop Hypertension- and Mediterranean-style dietary patterns and age-related cognitive change: the Cache County Study on Memory, Health and Aging. *Am J Clin Nutr.* 2013;98(5):1263-1271. doi:10.3945/ajcn.112.051276

3. Liu X, Dhana K, Barnes LL, et al. A healthy plant-based diet was associated with slower cognitive decline in African American older adults: a biracial community-based cohort. *Am J Clin Nutr.* 2022;116(4):875-886. doi:10.1093/ajcn/nqac204

4. USDA. Dietary Guidelines for Americans, 2020–2025. Accessed April 7, 2022. dietaryguidelines.gov/resources/2020-2025-dietary-guidelines-online-materials

5. Yeh TS, Yuan C, Ascherio A, Rosner BA, Blacker D, Willett WC. Long-term dietary protein intake and subjective cognitive decline in US men and women. *Am J Clin Nutr.* 2022;115(1):199-210. https://doi.org/10.1093/ajcn/nqab236

6. USDA. Dietary Guidelines for Americans, 2020–2025. Accessed April 7, 2022. dietaryguidelines.gov/resources/2020-2025-dietary-guidelines-online-materials

7. Chawla S, Tessarolo Silva F, Amaral Medeiros S, Mekary RA, Radenkovic D. The effect of low-fat and low-carbohydrate diets on weight loss and lipid levels: a systematic review and meta-analysis. *Nutrients.* 2020;12(12):3774. doi:10.3390/nu12123774

Chapter 12: Wine in Moderation

1. Stockley CS. Wine consumption, cognitive function and dementias—a relationship? *Nutr Aging.* 2015;3(2-4):125-137. doi:10.3233/NUA-150055

2. Braidy N, Jugder BE, Poljak A, et al. Resveratrol as a potential therapeutic candidate for the treatment and management of Alzheimer's disease. *Curr Top Med Chem.* 2016;16(17):1951-1960. doi:10.2174/1568026616666160204121431; Weiskirchen S, Weiskirchen R. Resveratrol: how much wine do you have to drink to stay healthy? *Adv Nutr Bethesda Md.* 2016;7(4):706-718. doi:10.3945/an.115.011627

3. Ilomaki J, Jokanovic N, Tan ECK, Lonnroos E. Alcohol consumption, dementia, and cognitive decline: an overview of systematic reviews. *Curr Clin Pharmacol.* 2015;10(3):204-212. doi:10.2174/1574884710003150820145539

4. Chao AM, Wadden TA, Tronieri JS, Berkowitz RI. Alcohol intake and weight loss during intensive lifestyle intervention for adults with overweight or obesity and diabetes. *Obesity.* 2019;27(1):30-40. doi:10.1002/oby.22316

Chapter 13: Saturated Fats: Red Meat, Butter, Cheese, Fried Foods, and Sweets

1. Wang DD, Li Y, Chiuve SE, et al. Association of specific dietary fats with total and cause-specific mortality. *JAMA Intern Med.* 2016;176(8):1134-1145. doi:10.1001/jamainternmed.2016.2417

2. Morris MC, Evans DA, Bienias JL, et al. Dietary fats and the risk of incident Alzheimer disease. *Arch Neurol.* 2003;60(2):194-200. doi:10.1001/archneur.60.2.194

3. USDA. Dietary Guidelines for Americans, 2020–2025. Accessed April 7, 2022. dietaryguidelines.gov/resources/2020-2025-dietary-guidelines-online-materials

4. Wang DD, Li Y, Chiuve SE, et al. Association of specific dietary fats with total and cause-specific mortality. *JAMA Intern Med.* 2016;176(8):1134-1145. doi:10.1001/jamainternmed.2016.2417

5. Schnaider Beeri M, Lotan R, Uribarri J, Leurgans S, Bennett DA, Buchman AS. Higher dietary intake of advanced glycation end products is associated with faster cognitive decline in community-dwelling older adults. *Nutrients.* 2022;14(7):1468. doi:10.3390/nu14071468

Chapter 14: MIND Diet FAQs: Lessons Learned from the Field

1. Morris MC, Tangney CC, Wang Y, et al. MIND diet slows cognitive decline with aging. *Alzheimers Dement.* 2015;11(9):1015-1022. doi:10.1016/j.jalz.2015.04.011

2. Malik VS, Hu FB. Sugar-sweetened beverages and cardiometabolic health: an update of the evidence. *Nutrients.* 2019;11(8):1840. doi:10.3390/nu11081840; Malik VS, Hu FB. Fructose and cardiometabolic health: what the evidence from sugar-sweetened beverages tells us. *J Am Coll Cardiol.* 2015;66(14):1615-1624. doi:10.1016/j.jacc.2015.08.025

3. AARP. Summer 2021 update to AARP's supplement survey. doi:10.26419/pia.00094.001

4. Baker LD, Manson JE, Rapp SR, et al. Effects of cocoa extract and a multivitamin on cognitive function: A randomized clinical trial. *Alzheimers Dement.* 2023;19(4):1308-1319. doi:10.1002/alz.12767

Chapter 15: Tools for Success

1. Ge L, Sadeghirad B, Ball GDC, et al. Comparison of dietary macronutrient patterns of 14 popular named dietary programmes for weight and cardiovascular

risk factor reduction in adults: systematic review and network meta-analysis of randomised trials. *BMJ.* 2020;369:m696. doi:10.1136/bmj.m696;

Shan Z, Wang F, Li Y, et al. Healthy eating patterns and risk of total and cause-specific mortality. *JAMA Intern Med.* 2023;183(2):142-153. doi:10.1001/jamainternmed.2022.6117

2. Teasdale N, Elhussein A, Butcher F, et al. Systematic review and meta-analysis of remotely delivered interventions using self-monitoring or tailored feedback to change dietary behavior. *Am J Clin Nutr.* 2018;107(2):247-256. doi:10.1093/ajcn/nqx048

3. Steptoe A. Happiness and health. *Annu Rev Public Health.* 2019;40(1):339-359. doi:10.1146/annurev-publhealth-040218-044150

4. Ryan RM, Deci EL. *Self-Determination Theory: Basic Psychological Needs in Motivation, Development, and Wellness.* Guilford Press; 2017:xii, 756. doi:10.1521/978.14625/28806

5. Bandura A. Self-efficacy: toward a unifying theory of behavioral change. *Psychol Rev.* 1977;84:191-215. doi:10.1037/0033-295X.84.2.191

6. Bandura A. *Social Foundations of Thought and Action: A Social Cognitive Theory.* Prentice-Hall; 1986:xiii, 617.

7. Christakis NA, Fowler JH. The spread of obesity in a large social network over 32 years. *N Engl J Med.* 2007;357(4):370-379. doi:10.1056/NEJMsa066082

Chapter 16: Tools for Weight Loss

1. Burke LE, Wang J, Sevick MA. Self-monitoring in weight loss: a systematic review of the literature. *J Am Diet Assoc.* 2011;111(1):92-102. doi:10.1016/j.jada.2010.10.008;

Ingels JS, Misra R, Stewart J, Lucke-Wold B, Shawley-Brzoska S. The effect of adherence to dietary tracking on weight loss: using HLM to model weight loss over time. *J Diabetes Res.* 2017;2017:1-8. doi:10.1155/2017/6951495;

Raber M, Liao Y, Rara A, et al. A systematic review of the use of dietary self-monitoring in behavioural weight loss interventions: delivery, intensity and effectiveness. *Public Health Nutr.* 2021;24(17):5885-5913. doi:10.1017/S13689 8002100358X

2. Ingels JS, Misra R, Stewart J, Lucke-Wold B, Shawley-Brzoska S. The effect of adherence to dietary tracking on weight loss: using HLM to model weight loss over time. *J Diabetes Res.* 2017;2017:1-8. doi:10.1155/2017/6951495

3. National Weight Control Registry. Accessed June 27, 2022. NWCR.ws

4. Burke LE, Wang J, Sevick MA. Self-monitoring in weight loss: a systematic review of the literature. *J Am Diet Assoc.* 2011;111(1):92-102. doi:10.1016/j.jada.2010.10.008

5. US Department of Veterans Affairs. Management of adult overweight and obesity. Accessed January 30, 2023. healthquality.va.gov/guidelines/CD/obesity/;

USDA. Dietary Guidelines for Americans, 2020–2025. Accessed April 7, 2022. dietaryguidelines.gov/resources/2020-2025-dietary-guidelines-online-materials

6. St-Onge MP, Ard J, Baskin ML, et al. Meal timing and frequency: implications for cardiovascular disease prevention: a scientific statement from the American Heart Association. *Circulation.* 2017;135(9):e96-e121. doi:10.1161/CIR.0000000000000476

7. Raynor HA, Epstein LH. Dietary variety, energy regulation, and obesity. *Psychol Bull.* 2001;127(3):325-341. doi:10.1037/0033-2909.127.3.325

8. St-Onge MP, Ard J, Baskin ML, et al. Meal timing and frequency: implications for cardiovascular disease prevention: a scientific statement from the American Heart Association. *Circulation.* 2017;135(9):e96-e121. doi:10.1161/CIR.0000000000000476

9. Bachman JL, Phelan S, Wing RR, Raynor HA. Eating frequency is higher in weight loss maintainers and normal weight individuals as compared to overweight individuals. *J Am Diet Assoc.* 2011;111(11):1730-1734. doi:10.1016/j.jada.2011.08.006

10. Varady KA, Cienfuegos S, Ezpeleta M, Gabel K. Clinical application of intermittent fasting for weight loss: progress and future directions. *Nat Rev Endocrinol.* 2022;18(5):309-321. doi:10.1038/s41574-022-00638-x;
St-Onge MP, Ard J, Baskin ML, et al. Meal timing and frequency: implications for cardiovascular disease prevention: a scientific statement from the American Heart Association. *Circulation.* 2017;135(9):e96-e121. doi:10.1161/CIR.0000000000000476

11. Raynor HA, Epstein LH. Dietary variety, energy regulation, and obesity. *Psychol Bull.* 2001;127(3):325-341. doi:10.1037/0033-2909.127.3.325

12. National Weight Control Registry. Accessed June 27, 2022. NWCR.ws;
Diabetes Prevention Program Research Group, Knowler WC, Fowler SE, et al. 10-year follow-up of diabetes incidence and weight loss in the Diabetes Prevention Program Outcomes Study. *Lancet Lond Engl.* 2009;374(9702):1677-1686. doi:10.1016/S0140-6736(09)61457-4;
Look AHEAD Research Group. Eight-year weight losses with an intensive lifestyle intervention: the look AHEAD study. *Obes Silver Spring Md.* 2014;22(1):5-13. doi:10.1002/oby.20662

Chapter 17: Your MINDful Life

1. Livingston G, Huntley J, Sommerlad A, et al. Dementia prevention, intervention, and care: 2020 report of the Lancet Commission. *Lancet Lond Engl.* 2020;396(10248):413-446. doi:10.1016/S0140-6736(20)30367-6

2. Steptoe A. Happiness and health. *Annu Rev Public Health.* 2019;40(1):339-359. doi:10.1146/annurev-publhealth-040218-044150

3. Chieffi S, Messina G, Villano I, et al. Exercise influence on hippocampal function: possible involvement of Orexin-A. *Front Physiol.* 2017;8:85. doi:10.3389/fphys.2017.00085

4. Baker LD, Cotman CW, Thomas R, et al. Topline results of EXERT: can exercise slow cognitive decline in MCI? *Alzheimer's Dement.* 2022;18:e069700. https://doi.org/10.1002/alz.069700

5. U.S. Department of Health and Human Services. Physical Activity Guidelines for Americans. Accessed May 27, 2023. Health.gov/our-work/nutrition-physical-activity/physical-activity-guidelines/current-guidelines

6. U.S. Department of Health and Human Services. Physical Activity Guidelines for Americans. Accessed May 27, 2023. Health.gov/our-work/nutrition-physical-activity/physical-activity-guidelines/current-guidelines

7. National Weight Control Registry. Accessed June 27, 2022. NWCR.ws

8. Lim ASP, Kowgier M, Yu L, Buchman AS, Bennett DA. Sleep fragmentation and the risk of incident Alzheimer's disease and cognitive decline in older persons. *Sleep*. 2013;36(7):1027-1032. doi:10.5665/sleep.2802

9. National Sleep Foundation. Sleep Statistics. Published May 18, 2023. Accessed May 27, 2023. thensf.org

10. Livingston G, Huntley J, Sommerlad A, et al. Dementia prevention, intervention, and care: 2020 report of the Lancet Commission. *Lancet Lond Engl*. 2020;396(10248):413-446. doi:10.1016/S0140-6736(20)30367-6

11. Livingston G, Huntley J, Sommerlad A, et al. Dementia prevention, intervention, and care: 2020 report of the Lancet Commission. *Lancet Lond Engl*. 2020;396(10248):413-446. doi:10.1016/S0140-6736(20)30367-6
Fowler JH, Christakis N. Dynamic spread of happiness in a large social network: longitudinal analysis over 20 years in the Framingham Heart Study. *Br Med J*. Published online 2008. doi:10.1136/bmj.a2338

12. Saito T, Murata C, Saito M, Takeda T, Kondo K. Influence of social relationship domains and their combinations on incident dementia: a prospective cohort study. *J Epidemiol Community Health*. 2018;72(1):7-12. doi:10.1136/jech-2017-209811

13. Bennett DA, Schneider JA, Buchman AS, Barnes LL, Boyle PA, Wilson SR. Overview and Findings from the Rush Memory and Aging Project. *Curr Alzheimer Res*. 2012;9(6):646-663. doi:10.2174/156720512801322663

14. Lloyd-Jones DM, Allen NB, Anderson CAM, et al. Life's essential 8: updating and enhancing the American Heart Association's construct of cardiovascular health: a presidential advisory from the American Heart Association. *Circulation*. 2022;146(5):e18-e43. doi:10.1161/CIR.0000000000001078

15. Livingston G, Huntley J, Sommerlad A, et al. Dementia prevention, intervention, and care: 2020 report of the Lancet Commission. *Lancet Lond Engl*. 2020;396(10248):413-446. doi:10.1016/S0140-6736(20)30367-6;
Lloyd-Jones DM, Allen NB, Anderson CAM, et al. Life's essential 8: updating and enhancing the American Heart Association's construct of cardiovascular health: a presidential advisory from the American Heart Association. *Circulation*. 2022;146(5):e18-e43. doi:10.1161/CIR.0000000000001078

16. Lewis NA, Turiano NA, Payne BR, Hill PL. Purpose in life and cognitive functioning in adulthood. *Neuropsychol Dev Cogn B Aging Neuropsychol Cogn*. 2017;24(6):662-671. doi:10.1080/13825585.2016.1251549

Chapter 18: 6 Weeks to a Healthy MIND

1. Hardcastle SJ, Thøgersen-Ntoumani C, Chatzisarantis NLD. Food choice and nutrition: a social psychological perspective. *Nutrients*. 2015;7(10):8712-8715. doi:10.3390/nu7105424

Appendix: The MIND Diet Program at a Glance and Sample Meal Plan

On the following pages you will find the "at a glance" version of the Official MIND Diet 6-Week Program. This can help you take a high-level look at the focus of each week, including the foods to track, a summary of small goals, and all the tools needed to complete the program. All that is left is your personal customization to make the program your own.

In addition you will find a 2-week sample meal plan for MIND diet eating. Good luck!

LEGEND

LG: leafy green vegetables
OV: other vegetables
Ber: berries
EVOO: extra-virgin olive oil
Nut: nuts & seeds

Fsh: fish & seafood
Poul: poultry
WG: whole grains
Bn: beans & legumes
Win: wine

RM: red meat & processed meat
But: butter & stick margarine
Chs: full-fat cheese
Fri: fried foods
Swt: sweets, pastries & sweet drinks

THE OFFICIAL MIND DIET 6-WEEK PROGRAM AT A GLANCE

6-Week SMART MIND Habits at a Glance

Week 1

Self-Monitoring	Meal Planning	Action Planning	Reflection	Trust & Support
Track all 15 MIND Foods **Tool:** MIND Diet Refrigerator Chart ***Weight Loss Bonus Tools/ Reminder:** Nutrition Tracking App and Body Weight Scale Be sure to calculate your 5% weight loss goal and record it in your journal.	**Schedule new habits of menu planning, grocery shopping, and meal preparation** in your Calendar. **Plan 1 menu item** for each day in your Calendar. **Tools/Reminder:** Be sure to add reminders to your Calendar as cues for you to engage in new habits.	**Small Goal #1:** Track all MIND diet foods without changing eating habits. Record your MIND Diet Score in your journal. **Small Goal #2:** Schedule 1 menu item each day without changing eating habits. **Tool/Reminder:** Be sure to make your small goals SMART and to post your Action Plan somewhere you will see it often.	**As you reflect on last week and each small goal, what were the successes? Barriers? How did you make your decisions?** **What was your MIND Diet Score?** **What was your experience with establishing a meal planning routine?** **Tool/Reminder:** Be sure to list 5 new things for which you feel grateful in your Reflection and Gratitude Journal.	**Tool/Reminder:** Scheduled time to meet with your Social Support Partner this week: _____

	Week 2			
Self-Monitoring	Meal Planning	Action Planning	Reflection	Trust & Support
Track Leafy Greens (LG), Other Vegetables (OV), Berries (Ber) + 5 Foods to Limit **Tool:** MIND Diet Refrigerator Chart ***Weight Loss Bonus Tools:** Nutrition Tracking App and Body Weight Scale	**Include LG, OV, and Ber as menu items for 1 meal each day in your Calendar.** **Create a grocery list and schedule a day to shop.** **Tools:** Calendar with Reminders, Menu Plan, grocery list	**Small Goal #1:** Track LG, OV, Ber, and the 5 Foods to Limit. **Small Goal #2:** Schedule LG, OV, and Ber into your menu. Make grocery list and go grocery shopping. **Tool/Reminder:** Be sure to make your Small Goals SMART. Consider adding a third MINDful life small goal if desired.	**What did you notice about your intake of the Foods to Limit this week?** **How sustainable do the meal planning activities of scheduling menu items and grocery shopping feel?** **Tool/Reminder:** Be sure to list 5 new things for which you feel grateful in your Reflection and Gratitude Journal.	**Tool/Reminder:** Scheduled time to meet with your Social Support Partner this week: _____

Week 3

Self-Monitoring	Meal Planning	Action Planning	Reflection	Trust & Support
Track Unsaturated Fats: Extra-Virgin Olive Oil (EVOO), Nuts & Seeds (Nut) + 5 Foods to Limit **Tool:** MIND Diet Refrigerator Chart ***Weight Loss Bonus Tools:** Nutrition Tracking App and Body Weight Scale	**Include EVOO and Nut as menu items for 1 meal each day in your Calendar.** **Identify recipes to enhance menu planning.** **Create a grocery list and schedule a day to shop.** **Tools:** Calendar with Reminders, Menu Plan, Recipe Bank, grocery list	**Small Goal #1:** Track EVOO, Nut, and the 5 Foods to Limit **Small Goal #2:** Schedule EVOO and Nut into your menu. Consider recipes in your menu plan. Make grocery list and schedule a day to shop. **Tool/Reminder:** Be sure to make your Small Goals SMART.	**How have your eating cues been influencing your food choices?** **How has your hydration been influencing your food choices?** **Describe your motivation to eat. Is it typically because you're hungry or for other reasons such as emotions, loneliness, boredom, when you are tired, or habitual mindless eating?** **Tool/Reminder:** Be sure to list 5 new things for which you feel grateful in your Reflection and Gratitude Journal.	**Tool/Reminder:** Scheduled time to meet with your Social Support Partner this week:

	Week 4			
Self-Monitoring	Meal Planning	Action Planning	Reflection	Trust & Support
Track Proteins: Fish & Seafood (Fsh), Poultry (Poul) + 5 Foods to Limit

Tool: MIND Diet Refrigerator Chart

*Weight Loss Bonus Tools: Nutrition Tracking App and Body Weight Scale | Include Fsh and Poul as menu items for 1 meal each day in your Calendar.

Identify recipes to enhance menu planning.

Create a grocery list and schedule a day to shop and meal prep.

Tools: Calendar with Reminders, Menu Plan, Recipe Bank, grocery list, meal prep plan

*Weight Loss Bonus Tool: Meal Timing Schedule | Small Goal #1: Track Fsh, Poul, and the 5 Foods to Limit.

Small Goal #2: Schedule Fsh and Poul into your menu. Consider recipes in your menu plan. Make grocery list, schedule a day to shop, meal prep for menu items up to 3 days ahead.

Tool/Reminder: Be sure to make your Small Goals SMART. | How does your environment impact your food choices?

How do the people around you influence your eating habits?

How do you think you're doing in the program so far? How confident do you feel in your ability to move forward?

How have things been going with your social support partner?

Tool/Reminder: Be sure to list 5 new things for which you feel grateful in your Reflection and Gratitude Journal. | Tool/Reminder: Scheduled time to meet with your Social Support Partner this week:

_____

*Weight Loss Bonus Tool: Lifestyle Program or Health Coach |

Week 5				
Self-Monitoring	Meal Planning	Action Planning	Reflection	Trust & Support
Track Carbohydrates: Whole Grains (WG), Beans/Legumes (Bn) + 5 Foods to Limit **Tool:** MIND Diet Refrigerator Chart ***Weight Loss Bonus Tools:** Nutrition Tracking App and Body Weight Scale	**Include WG and Bn as menu items for 1 meal each day in your Calendar.** **Identify recipes to enhance menu planning.** **Create a grocery list and schedule a day to shop, meal prep, and meal balance.** **Tools:** Calendar with Reminders, Menu Plan, Recipe Bank, grocery list, Meal Prep Plan, MIND Plate for Meal Planning ***Weight Loss Bonus Tool:** Meal Timing Schedule	**Small Goal #1:** Track WG, Bn, Win, and the 5 Foods to Limit. **Small Goal #2:** Schedule WG and Bn into your menu. Consider recipes in your menu plan. Make a grocery list, schedule a day to shop, meal prep for menu items up to 3 days ahead. Also consider using the MIND Plate for Meal Planning. **Tool/Reminder:** Be sure to make your Small Goals SMART.	**As you reflect on last week and each small goal, what were the successes? Barriers? How did you make your decisions?** **Describe how you feel after consuming the moderation foods (Win and 5 Foods to Limit) compared to when you have mostly plant-based, balanced meals.** **Tool/Reminder:** Be sure to list 5 new things for which you feel grateful in your Reflection and Gratitude Journal.	**Tool/Reminder:** Scheduled time to meet with your Social Support Partner this week: _____ ***Weight Loss Bonus Tool:** Lifestyle Program or Health Coach

Week 6

Self-Monitoring	Meal Planning	Action Planning	Reflection	Trust & Support
Track all 15 MIND Foods **Tool:** MIND Diet Refrigerator Chart ***Weight Loss Bonus Tools:** Nutrition Tracking App and Body Weight Scale	**Include Foods to Choose that need improvement and substitutions for Foods to Limit in your Calendar.** **Identify recipes to enhance menu planning.** **Create a grocery list and schedule a day to shop, meal prep, and meal balance.** **Tools:** Calendar with Reminders, Menu Plan, Recipe Bank, grocery list, meal prep plan, MIND Plate for Meal Planning ***Weight Loss Bonus Tool:** Meal Timing Schedule	**Small Goal #1:** Track all MIND Diet foods. Compare week 6 MIND Diet Score to week 1 MIND Diet Score. Record in your journal. **Small Goal #2:** Schedule Foods to Choose that need improvement in menu and find substitutes for Foods to Limit. Consider recipes in your menu plan. Make grocery list, schedule a day to shop, meal prep for menu items up to 3 days ahead. Also consider using the MIND Plate for Meal Planning.	**Review your past journal reflection entries from weeks 1-5.** **What motivated you to stay on track over the past 6 weeks?** **What made you feel energized over the past 6 weeks?** **What were your biggest successes over the past 6 weeks?** **What were your biggest barriers over the past 6 weeks?**	**Tool/Reminder:** Scheduled time to meet with your Social Support Partner this week: _____ ***Weight Loss Bonus Tool:** Lifestyle Program or Health Coach

SAMPLE 2-WEEK MEAL PLAN

Sample Meal Plan: Week 1

	Monday	Tuesday	Wednesday	Thursday	Friday	Saturday	Sunday
Breakfast	1 cup low-fat Greek yogurt ½ cup berries ½ cup whole-grain cereal or 2 tablespoons granola 2 tablespoons walnuts 1 tablespoon flax, chia, or hemp seeds (optional) **1 Ber, 1 Nut, 1 WG**	**Bonus Peanut Butter Toast** with boiled egg (optional) **1 Ber, 0.5 Nut, 1 WG**	1 cup low-fat Greek yogurt ½ cup berries ½ cup whole-grain cereal or 2 tablespoons granola 2 tablespoons walnuts 1 tablespoon flax, chia, or hemp seeds (optional) **1 Ber, 1 Nut, 1 WG**	Avocado Toast: Mix ½ smashed avocado, 1 tablespoon lemon juice, and a pinch cayenne pepper (optional). Serve on 2 slices whole-grain bread + 1 milk of choice **2 WG**	**Strawberry Green Breakfast Smoothie** **1 LG, 1 Ber, 1 Nut**	**Veggie Frittata** with whole-grain English muffin + 1 cup milk of choice **1.5 LG, 1 OV, 1 EVOO, 1 WG**	1 cup low-fat Greek yogurt 1 small apple sprinkled with cinnamon 2 tablespoons walnuts 1 tablespoon flax, chia, or hemp seeds (optional) **1 Nut**
Lunch	Turkey sandwich on whole-grain bread with low-fat cheese, mustard, lettuce, tomato. Side of baked chips, baby carrots, 2 tablespoons hummus **1 OV, 1 Poul, 2 WG, 0.5 Bn**	Kale or other leafy greens mixed with beets, bell peppers, edamame beans, tossed in 2 tablespoons **Regal Lemon-Shallot Dressing**, wrapped in whole-grain tortilla **1 LG, 1 OV, 0.5 EVOO, 1 WG**	Turkey sandwich on whole-grain bread with low-fat cheese, mustard, lettuce, tomato. Side of baked chips, baby carrots, 2 tablespoons hummus **1 OV, 1 Poul, 2 WG, 0.5 Bn**	**Chickpea Tuna Salad** on 1 slice whole-grain toast **0.5 OV, 1 EVOO, 0.5 Fsh, 1 WG, 0.5 Bn**	Tuna-avocado bites: Mix ¼ smashed avocado, 1 can tuna, 1½ teaspoons EVOO, ½ cup cooked brown rice, 1 tablespoon lemon juice, and a pinch cayenne pepper (optional). Serve with whole-grain crackers and bell peppers. **0.5 OV, 0.5 EVOO, 1 Fsh, 2 WG**	**Chickpea Tuna Salad** on 1 slice whole-grain toast **0.5 OV, 1 EVOO, 0.5 Fsh, 1 WG, 0.5 Bn**	Grilled chicken sandwich and cucumber-tomato salad with 1 tablespoon EVOO + balsamic vinegar + fresh basil **1 OV, 1 EVOO, 1 Poul**

Snack	2 tablespoons hummus + veggies **1 OV, 0.5 Bn**	Cucumber-tomato salad and ½ cup chickpeas with 1 tablespoon EVOO + balsamic vinegar + fresh basil **1 OV, 1 EVOO, 1 Bn**	1 slice whole-grain bread + 1 tablespoon EVOO **1 EVOO, 1 WG**	**Key Lime Smoothie** **1 LG**	1 cup low-fat Greek yogurt + small apple	1 high-fiber/high-protein granola bar	**Key Lime Smoothie** **1 LG**
Dinner	**Royal MIND Bowl** made with salmon + 1 glass red wine **1 LG, 1 OV, 0.5 Ber, 1 EVOO, 0.5 Nut, 1 Fsh, 1 WG, 1 Bn, 1 Win**	Leftover **Royal MIND Bowl** made with salmon + 1 glass red wine **1 LG, 1 OV, 0.5 Ber, 1 EVOO, 0.5 Nut, 1 Fsh, 1 WG, 1 Bn, 1 Win**	Stir-fry of chicken and broccoli, cauliflower, snowpeas, and bell peppers with **Soy-Sriracha Stir-Fry Sauce** over ½ cup brown rice **2 OV, 1 EVOO, 1 Poul, 1 WG**	Leftover stir-fry of chicken and broccoli, cauliflower, snowpeas, and bell peppers with **Soy-Sriracha Stir-Fry Sauce** over ½ cup brown rice **2 OV, 1 EVOO, 1 Poul, 1 WG**	2 slices homemade whole-grain pizza with **Arugula Hemp Seed Salad** **1 LG, 1 EVOO, 1 Nut, 2 WG, 1 Chs**	Dinner out: 1 red meat, 1 fried food, 2 desserts, + 1 glass red wine **1 RM, 1 Fri, 2 Swt, 1 Win**	Leftover 2 slices homemade whole-grain pizza with **Arugula Hemp Seed Salad** **1 LG, 1 EVOO, 1 Nut, 2 WG, 1 Chs**
Snack (Optional)	**2 Protein Power Bites** **0.5 Nut**		½ cup frozen berries **1 Ber**				½ cup frozen berries **1 Ber**

Provides Approximately: 1600–1800 Calories

Carb	40–45%
Protein	20–25%
Fat	30–35%
Sat. Fat	<10%

Sample Meal Plan: Week 2

	Monday	Tuesday	Wednesday	Thursday	Friday	Saturday	Sunday
Breakfast	Blueberry Pie Overnight Oats 1 Ber, 1 Nut, 1 WG	Blueberry Pie Overnight Oats 1 Ber, 1 Nut, 1 WG	Blueberry Pie Overnight Oats 1 Ber, 1 Nut, 1 WG	Spinach and Coffee Protein Smoothie with peanut butter toast 1 LG, 1 Nut, 1 WG	Spinach and Coffee Protein Smoothie with peanut butter toast 1 LG, 1 Nut, 1 WG	Olive Oil Veggie Scramble with 1 slice whole-grain toast 0.5 LG, 1 OV, 1 EVOO, 1 WG	Veggie Hash with Eggs 2 OV, 1 EVOO, 1 WG
Lunch	Lentil Quinoa Salad with Smoked Salmon and arugula with EVOO 1 LG, 1 OV, 2 EVOO, 0.5 Fsh, 1 WG, 1 Bn	Leftover Lentil Quinoa Salad with Smoked Salmon 1 OV, 1 EVOO, 1 Fsh, 1 WG, 1 Bn	3–5 ounces grilled chicken in whole-grain wrap with lettuce, tomato, Creamy Tahini Sauce, and Pickled Red Onions + 1 apple 1 LG, 1 OV, 1 Nut, 1 Poul, 1 WG	3–5 ounces grilled chicken in whole-grain wrap with lettuce, tomato, Creamy Tahini Sauce, and Pickled Red Onions + 1 orange 1 LG, 1 OV, 1 Nut, 1 Poul, 1 WG	2 pieces avocado toast with hard-boiled egg, salad of spinach, cucumber, and tomato + dressing of 1 tablespoon EVOO + 1 tablespoon balsamic vinegar + fresh herbs of choice 1 LG, 1 OV, 1 EVOO, 2 WG	Lunch out: cucumber/seaweed salad or miso soup, ½ order edamame, 1 order sushi roll 1 OV, 1 Fsh, 1 Bn	Warm Veggie Wrap 1 LG, 2.5 OV, 1 EVOO, 1 WG, 1 Bn
Snack	Carrot sticks and peanut butter 1 OV, 1 Nut	Spinach salad with hard-boiled egg, tomatoes, and **Goes with Everything Dressing** + whole-grain crackers 1 LG, 1 OV, 1.5 EVOO, 1 WG	**Spicy Black Bean Hummus** with whole-grain crackers 1 EVOO, 1 WG, 1 Bn	Spicy Black Bean Hummus with baked corn chips 1 EVOO, 1 WG, 1 Bn	Spicy Black Bean Hummus with bell peppers 1 OV, 1 EVOO, 1 WG, 1 Bn	Olive Oil Banana Bread with blueberries 1 Ber, 0.5 EVOO, 1 WG	Olive Oil Banana Bread with 1 tablespoon peanut butter 0.5 EVOO, 0.5 Nut, 1 WG

Dinner	Turkey Chili	Leftover Turkey Chili	Spaghetti Squash Bolognese	Spaghetti Squash Bolognese	Dinner out: Italian or Mediterranean	Crispy Fried Rice	Pasta with Marinated Tomatoes and Shrimp
	1.5 OV, 0.5 Poul, 0.5 Bn	1.5 OV, 0.5 Poul, 0.5 Bn	0.5 LG, 3 OV, 1 EVOO, 1 Poul	0.5 LG, 3 OV, 1 EVOO, 1 Poul	Dinner out: Italian or Mediterranean: leafy green salad with EVOO-based dressing, ½ plate vegetables, ¼ plate lean protein, ¼ plate whole grains if possible. Optional wine and shared dessert. 2 LG, 2 OV, 1 EVOO, 1 Fsh or Poul, 1 WG, 1 Win, 1 Swt	1 LG, 1.5 OV, 0.5 EVOO, 1 WG	and arugula salad with 1 tablespoon EVOO + dressing of 1 tablespoon lemon juice + fresh herbs of choice. 1 LG, 1 OV, 1 EVOO, 1 Fsh, 2 WG
Snack (Optional)	Olive Oil Popcorn 1 EVOO, 1 WG		1 ounce dark chocolate with 1 orange 1 Swt			Frozen berries and low-fat yogurt blended 1 Ber	

Provides Approximately:	
1600-1800 Calories	
Carb	40–45%
Protein	20–25%
Fat	30–35%
Sat. Fat	<10%

Index

Note: *Italic* page numbers refer to charts and illustrations.

accountability, 133–40, 167, 179–81, 183, 202
action-based goals, 160
Action Planning
  Small Goals List, 159–61, *161*, 162,
    163–65, 172, 191, 192, 201
  as SMART MIND habit, 132, 159–61, *161*,
    162, 163–65, 172, 201, *202*
  Week 1 and, 204–5, *204*
  Week 2 and, 210, *211*
  Week 3 and, *214*
  Week 4 and, 218–19, *218*
  Week 5 and, *227*
  Week 6 and, *231*
adenosine, 190
advanced glycation end products (AGEs),
  122–23
Agarwal, Puja, 41–42
Aggarwal, Neelum, 40
air fryers, 120
alcohol consumption. *See also* wine
  (Win)
  alcohol abuse symptoms, 15
  moderation of, 113–16, 159, 225, 228, 229
  sleep and, 190
  vitamin B_{12} levels and, 23
allergies, 84, 91, 93, 124, 219
alpha carotene, 35
alpha-linolenic acid (ALA), 84, 219
alternate-day fasting, 176
Alzheimer's Association, 20, 216
Alzheimer's disease
  beta-amyloid plaques and, 15–16, 20, 42, 62
  delayed onset of, 40
  diagnosis of, 15–16, 27, 29
  dietary fats and, 117
  genetic basis of, 6, 16
  increase in deaths from, 13
  lifestyle factors affecting, 16–17, 19, 31

MIND Diet Score and, 53–54, *54*
MIND Diet's reduction of risk of, 7, 17,
  28, 29, 35, 40, 41–42, 157
prevention of, 17, 25, 30, 32, 73
progression of, 6–7, 14
risk factors for, 19, 23, 27, 29, 35, *39*,
  41–42, 100, 125, 134, 230
sleep quality and, 189
social engagement and, 191
subjective cognitive decline and, 88
American Association of Retired People
  (AARP), 92
American Heart Association, 76–77, 89, 91,
  124, 173–74, 184
amino acids, 109
anthocyanin, 66, 72, 114
antioxidants
  carotenoids and, 24, 64
  extra-virgin olive oil and, 78, 80
  flavonols and, 41
  nuts and, 84
  vegetables and, 61, 64, 66
  vitamin E and, 20–21
  wine and, 114
Arugula Hemp Seed Salad, 86, 292–93
Arugula Pesto, 68, 314
atherosclerosis, 23
Autumn Roasted Vegetables with Apple
  Cider Sauce, 291–92
avocado toast, 103

Baker, Laura, 38, 39, 126, 183
Balsamic Berries, 303–4
Balsamic Reduction, 69, 81, 317–18
beans and legumes (Bn)
  carbohydrates and, 98, 106–10, *111*, 123,
    153
  Foods to Choose list, *57*

Index

as low advanced glycation end products foods, 123
MIND Diet Target, *107*
MIND Food Points, *111, 225*
MINDful bean swaps, 108–9
as protein source, 97, 98
bedtime routine, 190
behavioral techniques, 30
Bennett, David, 19
berries (Ber), *56*, 60, 72–75, *111*, 112, 114, 121, 153, 207
berry chutney, 74
berry syrup, 74
berry transfer, 75
berrywater, 74
beta-amyloid plaques, 15–16, 20, 42, 62, 78, 84, 114
beta-carotene, 24, 35, 61, 64, 66, 71
beverages. *See also* alcohol consumption
  berrywater, 74
  breakfast and, 174
  sugar-sweetened beverages, 112, 121, 125–26, 155, 159, 219, 220, 232
  water as, 65, 159, 179
  weight loss and, 179, 232–33
Black Americans, 102
Black Bean Veggie Burgers, 108, 277–79
blood-brain barrier, 23
blood pressure, 16, 31, 70, 91, 102, 107, 125, 185
Blueberry Pie Overnight Oats, 248–49
blue light, 191
body weight scale, 170–71, 206
Bonus Peanut Butter Toast, 103, 245–46
brain atrophy, 16, 113
brain-derived neurotrophic factor (BDNF), 183
brain health
  aging process and, 13–14, 21, 27, 32, 100
  beneficial nutrients affecting, 24–25
  berries and, 73
  essential nutrients affecting, 20–24
  MIND Diet's effect on, 26–29, 41, 42, 55, 170
  nutrition and, 6, 7, 8, 18, 19–20, 32
  optimization of, 59
  supplements for, 92, 126–27
  whole grains and, 100
breads, whole-grain breads, 102–3
breakfast, scheduling of, 173–74, 223
breakfast recipes
  Blueberry Pie Overnight Oats, 248–49
  Bonus Peanut Butter Toast, 245–46
  Chia Seed Pudding with Berries, 250
  Fancy Smoked Salmon Toast, 246–47
  Hippie Oat Bowls, 247–48

Key Lime Smoothie, 251
Loaded Breakfast Sandwich, 244–45
Olive Oil Veggie Scramble, 243–44
Spinach and Coffee Protein Smoothie, 252
Strawberry Green Breakfast Smoothie, 252–53
Veggie Frittata, 240–41
Veggie Hash with Eggs, 241–42
Brigham and Women's Hospital, Boston, 30
Broiled Arctic Char, 82, 90, 268–69
Buehner, Carl, 193
butter and stick margarine (But), *57, 77*, 118–19, *122*, 124, *138*, 155, 156
Butterfinger Bites, 309–10

caffeine, 190
Calendar with Reminders, 141–43, *142*, 161, 163, *203, 204,* 209
calories
  in alcohol, 115, 229
  in beverages, 232
  in carbohydrates, 99, 100, 101
  counting of, 49
  in dietary fats, 76
  eating cues and, 215
  in extra-virgin olive oil, 79, 80, 81, 155
  in *Foods to Limit,* 223
  intermittent fasting and, 176
  meal and snack frequency and, 175, 179
  on Nutrition Facts label, *147,* 148
  in nuts and seeds, 85, 86, 155
  in proteins, 88, 96–97, 153
  in saturated fats, 117, 119, 120
  sources of, 58–59
  traveling and restaurant meals and, 158
  weight loss and, 30, 61, 62, 65, 79, 86, 155, 229, 232
  in whole grains, 111
cancer, 117
canned fish, 90
Carb Manager, 169
carbohydrates
  beans and legumes (Bn), 98, 106–10, 111, 123, 153
  in berries, 73, 111
  complex carbohydrates, 99, 100
  as food category, 58, 73, 99
  low-fat diets and, 117
  as macronutrient, 58
  MIND Diet Targets, *100, 107*
  MIND Food Points, *111, 225*
  MIND Plate for Meal Planning and, 150, *150,* 151, *151,* 154
  simple carbohydrates, 99, 100
  total carbohydrates on Nutrition Facts label, 149

carbohydrates *(cont.)*
  in vegetables, 61
  Week 5 and, 225–29
  weight loss and, 103, 110–12
  in whole-grain breads, 103
  whole grains (WG), 99–106, 110, 111, 123,
    153
cardiovascular diseases
  beans and legumes and, 106
  DASH diet and, 27
  fatty fish and, 89
  meal and snack frequency and, 174
  meal timing and, 173
  Mediterranean diet and, 27
  MIND Diet's effect on, 42, 132
  monounsaturated fatty acids and, 78
  nuts and, 84
  physical activity and, 183
  refined carbohydrates and, 117
  risk factors for, 16, 38
  saturated fats and, 117
  sleep quality and, 189
  weight loss and, 172
carotenoids, 24, 61, 64
Carrot, Ginger, and Leek Soup, 279–80
Centers for Disease Control and Prevention,
    88
cheese, full-fat (Chs), *57, 77,* 118–20, *122,*
    124, *138,* 155–56
cherries, 125
Chewy Oatmeal Chocolate Chip Cookies,
    312–13
Chia Seed Pudding with Berries, 86, 250
Chicago Health and Aging Project (CHAP),
    19, 20, 26, 55, 72–73, 78, 93
Chickpea Skillet Bars, 310–11
Chickpea Tuna Salad, 82, 90, 108, 144,
    273
cholesterol, on Nutrition Facts label, 148
cholesterol levels
  alcohol consumption and, 115
  dementia risks and, 31
  dietary cholesterol and, 124–25
  fiber and, 111
  management of, 16, 23, *77,* 78, 89, 110,
    119, 125
  saturated fats and, 120, 125
  whole grains and, 102
circadian rhythms, 175, 190–91
citrus, 70, 123, 154
coconut oil, 126
cognitive decline
  advanced glycation end products and,
    122, 123
  aging process and, 14, 27, 100
  alcohol consumption and, 114

beans and legumes and, 106
berries and, 72
fish and seafood and, 89
lifestyle practices and, 38
MIND Diet Score and, 54
MIND Diet's effect on, 29, 31, 35, 40, 41,
    102, 132, 157
prevention of, 27, 29
risk factors for, 16, 126
saturated fats and, 117, 118, 120–21
seafood consumption and, 21
subjective cognitive decline, 88
vitamin B levels and, 93
vitamin E levels and, 20
cognitive engagement, 39
cognitive functioning
  intellectual engagement and, 193–94
  leafy green vegetables and, 62
  Mind Diet's effect on, 35, 37, 41, 101–2
  multidomain lifestyle approach and, 38
  nuts and, 84
  other vegetables and, 64
  proteins and, 88
  whole grains and, 100, 101
cognitive processing, speed of, 14, 64
cognitive reserve theory, 191
cooking methods
  advanced glycation end products and,
    122–23
  extra-virgin olive oil and, 79–80
  feeling like you "don't cook," 144–45
  high-heat cooking, 80, 123
  traveling and restaurant meals and, 158
Covey, Stephen, 140
COVID-19 pandemic, 32, 34, 35, 36
Creamy Spinach Dip, 68, 298–300
Creamy Tahini Sauce, 68, 69, 316
Crispy Brussels Sprouts with Savory Sauce,
    287–88
Crispy Fried Rice, 282–84
"crunch-salty" flavors, 67–68
cultural traditions, 48, 124, 132, 230
Curried Coconut Vegetable Stew, 284–85

dairy products, 55, 124–25
DASH (Dietary Approaches to Stop
    Hypertension) diet
  MIND Diet compared to, 28–29, 40
  poultry consumption and, 93
  sodium intake and, 126
  studies on, 27
  whole grains and, 101, 106
dehydration, 15, 215
dementia. *See also* Alzheimer's disease
  alcohol consumption and, 113
  diagnosis of, 13–15

dietary links and, 19, 20
lifestyle practices and, 38
Martha Clare Morris's research on, 6–8, 33
prevention of, 16–17, 19, 24, 38, 159
randomized dietary intervention trial for, 7–9, 26–29
risk factors for, 16, 29, 31, 38
subjective cognitive decline and, 88
types of, 14
depression, 15, 89
DHA (docosahexaenoic acid), 21–22, 89, 92, 219
diabetes
advanced glycation end products and, 122
alcohol consumption and, 115, 116
fasting and, 177
MIND Diet's effect on, 42
prevention and management program for, 169
reducing risk for, 125
saturated fats and, 120
type 2 diabetes, 115, 117, 174
weight loss and, 172
whole grains and, 102
dietary fats. *See also* saturated fats; trans fats; unsaturated fats
controversy on, 117–18
fat swaps, *121*
function of, 76, *77*
as macronutrient, 58
MIND Plate for Meal Planning and, 150, *150*, 151, *151*, 155–56
total fat on Nutrition Facts label, 148
types of, 23–24
in vegetables, 61
Dietary Guidelines for Americans (2020–2025), 102, 106, 117
dietary restrictions, 124
Diet for the MIND (Martha Clare Morris), 8, 41
diet industry, 41
digestive enzymes, 58
DNA damage, 24–25
dried berries, 74
drug interactions, 15
drug use, 15

eating habits. *See* Self-Monitoring
EatRight.org, 180
edamame, 109
eggs, 23, 55, 63, 75, 97, 124–25
electronics, 190–91
emotional health and well-being, 15, 89
Environmental Protection Agency, 91

exercise. *See also* movement; physical activity
aerobic exercises, 184, 185–86, 188–89
anaerobic exercises, 184, 185, 186
creating habit of, 187
FITT principle for, 184–85, 186
EXERT trial, 183
extra-virgin olive oil (EVOO), 56, 76, 77–83, 105, 118, 119, 126
extrinsic motivation, 164

Fancy Smoked Salmon Toast, 90, 103, 246–47
Farro and Arugula Salad, 294–95
fat-soluble vitamins, 5
fiber
beans and legumes and, 107, 112
berries and, 73, 125
as carbohydrate, 111, 112
insoluble fiber, 99
leafy green vegetables and, 61–62
other vegetables and, 65
soluble fiber, 99
whole grains and, 100, 101, 103, 112
Fiesta Chopped Salad, 296–97
FINGER (Finnish Geriatric Intervention Study to Prevent Cognitive Impairment and Disability) trial, 38–39
fish and seafood (Fsh)
allergies to, 91, 93
avoidance of, 91–93
fatty fish, 82, 89, 92, 118, 119, 154
Foods to Choose list, 56
MIND Plate for Meal Planning and, 153
proteins and, 89–93, 96, 97
fish oil supplements, 21–22, 92
flavonoids, 25, 61, 72, 73
flavonols, 41
folate, 22, 23, 61, 100, 106
folate supplements, 22
food allergies, 84, 91, 93, 124, 219
Food and Drug Administration, 91
food availability, 48
food intolerances, 48
food labels, 146–47, *147*
food preferences, 48–49, 91, 124, 132, 230
free radicals, 23, 24, 125
fried foods (Fri)
beta-amyloid load and, 42
Foods to Limit list, 58, 77, 111–12, 118, 120, *138*, 155, 156, 158, *209*, 230
MIND Food Points, *122*
Reflection and, 215, 219
frozen berries, 74–75
frozen fish, 90–91
frozen meals, 71, 110

frozen poultry, 94
frozen veggies, 71
fruit. *See also* vegetables and fruit
 berries, 56, 60, 72–75, 111, 112, 114, 121, 125, 153
 carbohydrates in, 73, 111
 MIND Diet Target, *72*
 sugars in, 125
fullness, feeling of, 62, 65, 96–97, 107, 111

Garlicky Yogurt Sauce, 68, 81, 315
global cognition, 102
Global Council on Brain Health (GCBH), 92
glucose, 99, 101, 176, 177
gluten intolerance or sensitivities, 106
goals. *See also* Small Goals List
 action-based goals, 160
 growth over goals mindset, 187
 long-term goals, 159, 161
Goes with Everything Dressing, 63, 69, 81, 94, 318–19
gratitude
 gratitude list, 165, 206, 227
 practice of, 196, 221
 Reflection and Gratitude Journal, 162–65, 201, *205*, 231
Grilled Chicken Spiedies, 95, 256–57
grocery delivery services, 146
grocery lists, 146
grocery shopping
 for extra-virgin olive oil, 80
 for frozen meals, 71
 Meal Planning and, 145–50, 204, 210
 for nuts and seeds, 85, 87
 Week 1 and, 204
 Week 2 and, 210, 211
 Week 3 and, 214
 Week 6 and, 230
 for whole grains, 101, *101*, 102–3
growth over goals mindset, 187

habits. *See* Action Planning; *In a Routine* foods; *In a Rush* foods; Meal Planning; Reflection; Self-Monitoring; SMART MIND habits; Trust and Support
happiness, 194–97, 234
Harvard T. H. Chan School of Public Health, 18, 27, 30
HDL cholesterol, 23, *77*, 110, 115, 119
health metrics, self-monitoring of, 39
Health Professionals Follow-Up Study, 88, 118
heart health, 59. *See also* cardiovascular diseases
high blood pressure, 31, 70, 91, 102, 107, 125
Hill, James O., 170
Hippie Oat Bowls, 86, 104, 247–48

hippocampus, 15, 183
Holland, Thomas, 41
homocysteine levels, 22, 23
hunger level, 216
hydration, 214–15
hydrogenated oils, 23, *77*

In a Routine foods
 beans and legumes, 107–9
 berries and, 74–75
 extra-virgin olive oil, 81–82
 fish and seafood, 90
 leafy green vegetables and, 62–63
 nuts and seeds, 85
 other vegetables, 66–70
 poultry, 94–95
 whole grains, 102–4
In a Rush foods
 beans and legumes, 109–10
 berries, 75
 breakfast and, 174
 extra-virgin olive oil, 82–83
 fish and seafood, 90–91
 leafy green vegetables, 64
 nuts and seeds, 86–87
 other vegetables, 70–71
 poultry, 95
 whole grains, 104–5
inflammation
 advanced glycation end products and, 122
 beans and legumes and, 106
 flavonoids and, 25
 homocysteine levels and, 22, 23
 saturated fats and, 117, 157
 sleep quality and, 189
 whole grains and, 106
insomnia, 189
insulin resistance, 117
intellectual engagement, 182, 193–94, 234
intermittent fasting (IF), 132, 175–78, 224
intrinsic motivation, 164, 165–66, 181
iron-deficiency anemia, 72

journaling, Reflection and Gratitude Journal, 162–65, 201, *205*, 231
junk food, veggies made to mimic, 67–68

Keller, Helen, 165
Key Lime Smoothie, 64, 174, 251
kidney disease, 122
Kivipelto, Miia, 39

lactation, 177
late-night eating, 175, 224
LDL cholesterol, 23, *77*, 78, 89, 110, 119
lean body mass, 96, 97

Lentil Quinoa Salad with Smoked Salmon, 274–75
leptin, 62, 65
lettuce wraps, 63
Lewy body dementia, 14–15
lifestyle practices
    happiness and, 194–97, 234
    integration of MIND Diet and, 43, 49
    lifestyle program or health coach, 179–81, 224
    movement and, 9, 16
    multidomain lifestyle approach and, 38–39
    physical activity and, 182–88
    sleep and, 9, 182, 189–91, 234
    social engagement and, 9, 182, 191–94, 234
    sustainability of, 161, 212
Loaded Breakfast Sandwich, 244–45
long-term goals, 159, 161
Look AHEAD study, 115
Lose It, 169
low-carbohydrate diets, 110, 117–18, 132
low-fat diets, 110, 117
lupini beans, 109
lutein, 24, 35, 61
lycopene, 66, 71

macronutrients, 58–59, 61, 76
main meal recipes
    Black Bean Veggie Burgers, 277–79
    Broiled Arctic Char, 268–69
    Carrot, Ginger, and Leek Soup, 279–80
    Chickpea Tuna Salad, 273
    Crispy Fried Rice, 282–84
    Curried Coconut Vegetable Stew, 284–85
    Grilled Chicken Spiedies, 256–57
    Lentil Quinoa Salad with Smoked Salmon, 274–75
    MIND Diet Board, 263–65
    Pasta with Marinated Tomatoes and Shrimp, 271–72
    Poached Salmon with Toasted Almonds and Parsley, 270–71
    Rice Noodles with Stir-Fried Vegetables, 280–82
    Roast Chicken, 265–66
    Royal MIND Bowls, 261
    Saturday Stew, 259–60
    Smoked Paprika Chicken with Seared Green Beans, 257–58
    Spaghetti Squash Bolognese, 267–68
    Turkey Chili, 262–63
    Turkish Tabbouleh with Chicken Meatballs, 254–56
    Warm Veggie Wrap, 285–86
    White Fish with Olives and Artichokes, 275–77

margarine. *See* butter and stick margarine (But)
marinades, 81, 123
Meal Planning
    Calendar with Reminders, 141–43, *142*, 161, 163, 203–4, *203*, 209
    grocery shopping and, 145–50, 204, 210
    Meal Preparation Plan, 149–50, 204, 230
    meal timing schedule, 173–79, *178*
    Menu Plan and, 143–45, 204, 211, 214, 218, 226, 230
    MIND Plate for Meal Planning, 150–57, *150*, *151*
    Recipe Bank and, 143–45
    Small Goals List and, 159
    as SMART MIND habit, 62, 132, 140–59, 201, *202*
    Week 1 and, 203–7
    Week 2 and, 209–10
    Week 3 and, 213–14
    Week 4 and, 218
    Week 5 and, 226
    Week 6 and, 230
meal timing schedule, 173–79, *178*, 222, 223–24
measurable goals, 160
Mediterranean diet
    Alzheimer's disease pathology and, 42
    extra-virgin olive oil and, 77
    fish consumption and, 89
    MIND Diet compared to, 28–29, 40
    nuts and, 84
    poultry consumption and, 93
    randomized dietary intervention trial and, 27, 28
    whole grains and, 101, 106
Mediterranean restaurants, 158
Meetup.com, 167
melatonin, 90, 191
memory
    Alzheimer's disease and, 15
    cognitive decline and, 14
    complex carbohydrates and, 100
    episodic memory, 102
    fish and seafood and, 90
    flavonoids and, 25
    long-term memory function, 183
    vitamin B_{12} and, 22
Memory and Aging Project (MAP) study
    advanced glycation end products and, 123
    berries and, 72–73
    brain tissue analysis and, 19–20, 41–42
    evidence gathered by, 26, 41, 55
    extra-virgin olive oil and, 78
    leafy green vegetables and, 62

Memory and Aging Project study *(cont.)*
 MIND Diet Score and, 7–8, 27–29, 35, 40,
  53–54
 Martha Clare Morris and, 19–20, 189
 seafood consumption and, 21
 stroke history and, 40
 vitamin D and cognitive performance
  and, 25
Menu Plan, 143–45, 204, 211
mercury levels, 21, 91–92
mild cognitive impairment (MCI), 14, 183
MIND Center for Brain Health, Rush
  University Medical Center, 33
MIND (Mediterranean-DASH Intervention
  for Neurodegenerative Delay) Diet.
  See also Official MIND Diet 6-Week
  Program; SMART MIND habits
 Alzheimer's disease prevention and, 17
 choices in, 43, 49, 55, 112, 113, 118, 120,
  121, 132, 147, 157, 161, 181, 201, 229
 dietary intervention trial for dementia and,
  7–9, 26–29, 30, 31–32, 33, 34–37, 38, 40,
  41, 92, 172, 180
 FAQs, 124–27
 FINGER trial and, 38–39
 Foods to Choose list, 42, 43, *55–57, 77*, 114,
  117, 126, *136*, 150, 169, 170, 203, *208,*
  209, 210, 220, 230, 231
 Foods to Limit list, 42, 43, 55, *57–58, 77*, 111,
  117, 118–21, 123, 125–26, *138*, 150, 155–57,
  158, 169, 203, 207, *208–9*, 209, 210–11,
  215, 217, 220, 223, 225, 227, 230, 231
 how to eat emphasized in, 87, 134, 147
 multidomain lifestyle approach and,
  38–39, 49
 protection against cognitive decline and, 40
 protection against neurodegenerative
  diseases and, 26
 ranking of diets and, 42
 research-based foundation of, 49, 124
 studies of, 102
 toolbox for, 42–43, 132, *133*
MIND Diet Board, 263–65
MIND Diet Quiz, 50–51, *51–53*, 54, 203, 233
MIND Diet Refrigerator Chart
 Self-Monitoring, 134–35, *135, 136–39*,
  156–57, 159, 163, 169–71, 179, 201, 202, 203
 Week 1 and, 203, 205–6
 Week 2 and, 208, 212
 Week 3 and, 217
 Week 4 and, 222, 223
 Week 5 and, 225
 Week 6 and, 230, *231*
MIND Diet Score
 balancing of, 112, 156–57
 interpretation of, 53–55

long-term goals and, 159
 MIND Diet Quiz and, 50–53
 plant-based foods and, 132
 randomized dietary intervention trial
  and, 27–29, 35–36
 recording of, 201, 202
 risk reductions and, *54*, 84
 Week 1 and, 202, 203, 205
 Week 2 and, 210
 Week 6 and, 230
MIND foods, weekly tracking of, 112
MINDful eating strategies, 30, 66
MIND meals, balancing of, 112
MIND Plate for Meal Planning, 150–57, *150,
  151*, 225, 226
mindset, 135, 162, 165, 166, 187, 220
moderation foods, 113–14, 118, 156, 157,
  227, 228, 229, 232
monounsaturated fats, 23, *77*, 82, 118, 119,
  121, *121*
monounsaturated fatty acids (MUFAs),
  78
Morris, Clare, 4, 5
Morris, Laura
 family life of, 4–5, 6, 237–39
 professional career of, 8, 49, 237–38
Morris, Martha Clare
 dementia research of, 6–9, 33
 on dietary fats, 117
 on effects of diet among other lifestyle
  factors, 39
 on food as medicine, 4, 5, 9
 illness and death of, 8, 31–32, 34
 MIND Diet created by, 27, 39, 40–41,
  48
 as nutritional epidemiologist, 4–6, 18–19,
  26–29, 33–34, 36–37, 38, 48
 on physical activity, 182–83
 on positive outlook, 194–95
 on scientific process, 3–4, 55
 on sleep quality, 189
 on social engagement, 191
 on supplement studies, 92
 on testing MIND Diet and lifestyle
  practices, 39–40
motivation, 164, 165–66, 202, 215, 227
movement, 9, 14–15, 16, 187. *See also*
  exercise; physical activity
multivitamin supplements, 126–27
myelin, 22–23
MyFitnessPal, 169
MyNetDiary, 169

National Health and Nutrition Examination
  Survey (NHANES 2011–2014), 88
National Institute on Aging, 29, 40

National Institutes of Health (NIH), 20, 29, 31
National Sleep Foundation, 189
National Weight Control Registry (NWCR), 170, 173, 180, 188
Netherlands study, 64
neural reserve, 193
neurodegenerative diseases, 26–29
neurofibrillary tangles, 15, 16, 20, 42
neurons, 15, 16, 21, 113
neuroplasticity, 183
niacin, 93
nondiet approach, 49
Nurses' Health Study, 72, 88, 106, 118
nut bars, 87
nut butters, 83, 85, 86–87
Nutrition Facts label, 147–49, *147*
nutrition tracking app, 168–70, 171, 206–7, 212, 216, 222, 233
nuts and seeds (Nut), *56*, 76, 83–87, 118, 121

oatmeal, 74, 75, 99, 100, 102, 104
obesity
    alcohol consumption and, 115, 116
    breakfast skipping and, 173
    dementia risk and, 31
    meal and snack frequency and, 174–75
    MIND Diet's effect on, 42
    reducing risk for, 125
    refined carbohydrates and, 117
    saturated fats and, 120
    vitamin D and, 25
Official MIND Diet 6-Week Program. *See also* SMART MIND habits
    customization of, 59, 124, 132, 141, 161, 163, 177, 181, 182, 190, 195–97, 201, 204, 210, 224, 229–30, 263–64, 337
    goals for, 161, 233
    journaling and, 162–65, 201, *205*, 231
    overview of, 337–43
    purpose of, 43, 49
    sample meal plans, 229, 344–47
    sleep and, 190–91, 234
    social support partners and, 166–67
    timeframe of, 160
    tools for, 131–33
    Week 1, 202–7, 338
    Week 2, 207–12, 339
    Week 3, 213–17, 340
    Week 4, 217–24, 341
    Week 5, 225–29, 342
    Week 6, 229–34, 343
    weight loss and, 172–73
Olive Oil Banana Bread, 304–5
Olive Oil Popcorn, 105, 301–2

Olive Oil Veggie Scramble, 144, 243–44
omega-3 fatty acids
    as essential nutrient for brain health, 21–22
    in fatty fish, 89, 92, 119
    nuts as source of, 84
    supplements for, 92, 126, 219
optimism, 195–96
osteoporosis, 25
oxidative stress, 24, 122

Parkinson's disease, 15
Pasta with Marinated Tomatoes and Shrimp, 90, 271–72
pelargonidin, 42, 73
perceptual speed, 102
phosphorylated tau tangles, 42, 73
physical activity. *See also* exercise; movement
    accepting changes and, 187–88
    alcohol consumption and, 115–16
    FITT principle for, 184–85, *186*
    frequency of, 184, 224
    growth over goals mindset, 187
    intensity of, 184, *185*
    lifestyle practices and, 182–88
    multidomain lifestyle approach and, 39
    strategies for, 186–87
    type of, 185–86
    weight loss and, 185, 188–89, 222, 224
Physical Activity Guidelines for Americans, 184
phytochemicals, 61
Pickled Red Onions, 320–21
plant-based meat alternatives, 219
Poached Salmon with Toasted Almonds and Parsley, 90, 270–71
polyphenols, 5, 24–25, 78, 84, 114, 154
polyunsaturated fats, 23, 82, 89, 118, 119, 121, *121*
polyunsaturated fatty acids (PUFAs), 80
portions
    beans and legumes and, 107
    berries and, 75
    carbohydrates and, 111–12
    definition of, 152
    extra-virgin olive oil and, 79, 82, 155
    hands used for estimating, *151*, 152–53
    moderation foods and, 156
    nuts and seeds and, 84, 85, 86, 155
    serving size distinguished from, 151–52
    snack foods and, 215
    weight loss and, 30
    whole grains and, 102
positive thinking, 196
poultry (Poul), *56*, 93–95, 96, 97, 119, 153

PREDIMED study, 84
pregnancy, 22, 177
Protein Power Bites, 86, 308–9
proteins
    beans and legumes and, 107, 109
    fish and seafood, 89–93, 96, 97
    as macronutrient, 58, 88
    MIND Diet Targets, 89, 93
    MIND Food Points, 96, 217
    MIND Plate for Meal Planning and, 150,
        150, 151, 151, 153, 154
    on Nutrition Facts label, 149
    plant sources of, 97, 219
    poultry, 56, 93–95, 96, 97, 119, 153
    in vegetables, 61
    Week 4 and, 217–24
    weight loss and, 96–98, 112
Pumpkin Pie Parfaits, 305–7
purpose in life, 196–97

rate of perceived exertion (RPE), 184, 185
realistic goals, 160
Recipe Bank, 143–45
red meat and processed meat (RM), 57, 77,
    118–19, 122, 138, 155, 156, 208, 230
refined grains, 99, 100
Reflection
    Reflection and Gratitude Journal, 162–65,
        201, 205, 231
    as SMART MIND habit, 132, 161–65, 201,
        202
    Week 1 and, 205–6
    Week 2 and, 210–11
    Week 3 and, 214–16
    Week 4 and, 219–21
    Week 5 and, 227
    Week 6 and, 229, 231
Regal Lemon-Shallot Dressing, 63, 69, 94,
    319–20
registered dietitians, 180, 224
religious traditions, 48
REM (rapid eye movement) sleep, 190
restaurant meals, tips for healthy eating,
    157–59
resveratrol, 114
retina, DHA in, 21
Rice Noodles with Stir-Fried Vegetables,
    280–82
Roast Chicken, 95, 265–66
Roasted Kale Chips, 297–98
Roosevelt, Eleanor, 197
rotisserie chicken, 95
Royal MIND Bowls, 261
Rush University Medical Center, 7, 8, 19,
    30, 40, 41, 48, 101–2

Sacks, Frank, 27
salads. *See also* sides, salads, and snacks
        recipes
    beans and legumes and, 107, 108
    as main course, 62
    poultry and, 94, 95
    salad dressings, 81
    salad kits, 64
    for traveling and restaurant meals, 158
    weekly salad prep, 67
    weekly salads, 63
sample meal plans, 229, 344–47
satiety hormones, 62, 65, 96, 98, 107, 179
saturated fats
    in butter, 23, 119
    in cheese, 23, 119–20
    consumption of, 117–21, 124, 125, 155–57
    fat swaps, 121
    in frozen meals, 110
    function of, 77
    MIND Diet Targets, 118
    MIND Food Points, 122
    substitutions for, 82
Saturday Stew, 259–60
sauces and toppers recipes
    Arugula Pesto, 314
    Balsamic Reduction, 317–18
    Creamy Tahini Sauce, 316
    Garlicky Yogurt Sauce, 315
    Goes with Everything Dressing, 318–19
    Pickled Red Onions, 320–21
    Regal Lemon-Shallot Dressing, 319–20
    Soy-Sriracha Stir-Fry Sauce, 317
    Toasted Nuts, 321–22
Sautéed Greens, 290
Savory Almond Corn on the Cob, 288–89
seafood. *See* fish and seafood (Fsh)
self-determination theory, 164
self-efficacy, 165–66
Self-Monitoring
    MIND Diet Refrigerator Chart, 134–35,
        135, 136–39, 156–57, 159, 163, 169–71,
        179, 201, 202, 203
    nutrition tracking app, 168–70
    as SMART MIND habit, 132, 133–40,
        201, 202
    Week 1 and, 203
    Week 2 and, 208–9
    Week 3 and, 213
    Week 4 and, 217–18
    Week 5 and, 225
    Week 6 and, 230
    weight loss and, 171, 172–73, 212
self-talk, 196
self-trust, 165–66, 181, 201, 221

serotonin, 90, 93
serving sizes
  definition of, 152
  on Nutrition Facts label, 148
  portions distinguished from, 151–52
  Week 1 and, 203
7 Habits of Highly Effective People, The
  (Covey), 140
sides, salads, and snacks recipes
  Arugula Hemp Seed Salad, 292–93
  Autumn Roasted Vegetables with Apple
    Cider Sauce, 291–92
  Creamy Spinach Dip, 298–300
  Crispy Brussels Sprouts with Savory
    Sauce, 287–88
  Farro and Arugula Salad, 294–95
  Fiesta Chopped Salad, 296–97
  Olive Oil Popcorn, 301–2
  Roasted Kale Chips, 297–98
  Sautéed Greens, 290
  Savory Almond Corn on the Cob, 288–89
  Spicy Black Bean Hummus, 300–301
  Tuscan Kale Salad, 293–94
sleep
  eating patterns and, 175
  lifestyle practices and, 9, 182, 189–91, 234
  weight loss and, 191
sleep apnea, 189
sleep disturbance, 189–91
sleep environment, 190
slow cookers, 94
Small Goals List
  Action Planning, 159–61, *161*, 162,
    163–65, 172, 191, 192, 201
  Week 1 and, 204–5, *204*
  Week 2 and, 210, *211*
  Week 3 and, *214*
  Week 4 and, *218*
  Week 5 and, 227, *227*
  Week 6 and, *231*
SMART MIND habits
  Action Planning, 132, 159–61, *161*, 162,
    163–65, 172, 201, *202*
  Meal Planning, 62, 132, 140–59, 201, *202*
  Reflection, 132, 161–65, 201, *202*
  Self-Monitoring, 132, 133–40, 201, *202*
  SMART MIND toolbox for success,
    42–43, 132, *133*
  Trust and Support, 132, 165–67, 201, *202*
Smoked Paprika Chicken with Seared
  Green Beans, 257–58
snack foods. *See also* sides, salads, and
  snacks recipes
  beans and legumes and, 109
  berries and, 75

carbohydrates and proteins combined in,
  104, 109, 149, 158
meal timing and, 178, 223
nuts and seeds and, 85, 86, 87
portions and, 215
traveling and, 158
veggie snacks, 66, 67–68
weight loss and, 170
whole grains and, 83, 104, 105
social cognitive theory, 166
social engagement
  guidelines for, 192–93, 194
  lifestyle practices and, 9, 182, 191–94, 234
  multidomain lifestyle approach and, 39
social groups, influence on eating habits,
  220–21
social isolation, 192
social media, 166, 195–96
social support partners
  accountability and, 183, 202
  Reflection and, 162
  Trust and Support and, 166–67
  Week 1 and, 206
  Week 2 and, 211–12
  Week 3 and, 216
  Week 4 and, 221–22
  Week 5 and, 228
  Week 6 and, 232
  weight loss and, 181
sodium
  in butter, 119
  in canned beans and legumes, 107
  in canned or frozen fish and seafood, 91
  in cheese, 119
  in frozen meals, 71
  healthful range of, 126
  low-sodium soy sauce, 68, 69, 70, 81, 109
  on Nutrition Facts label, 148–49
  roasted chickpeas, 109–10
  in seasonings, 94
  in vegetable juices, 66
  in whole-grain breads, 103
Soy-Sriracha Stir-Fry Sauce, 63, 317
Spaghetti Squash Bolognese, 95, 267–68
specific goals, 160
spices, 69, 70, 81
Spicy Black Bean Hummus, 68, 108,
  300–301
Spinach and Coffee Protein Smoothie, 64,
  252
Strawberry Green Breakfast Smoothie, 64,
  86, 174, 252–53
stress, reduction of, 16
stroke survivors, 40
subjective cognitive decline (SCD), 88

sugars
  beverages and, 112, 121, 125–26, 155, 159,
    219, 220, 232
  as carbohydrate, 111
  limiting intake of, 120–21, 125–26
  low-fat diets and, 117
  processed grains associated with, 99, 100
  sugar swaps, *122*
  in whole-grain breads, 103
support. *See also* social support partners;
    Trust and Support
  lifestyle program or health coach for,
    179–81, 222, 224
  personal trainers and, 183
sweets, pastries, and sweet drinks (Swt)
  beta-amyloid load and, 42
  Foods to Limit list, *58, 77,* 111–12, 120–21,
    125–26, *138,* 155, *209,* 210
  MIND Food Points, *122*
  Reflection and, 219
  Self-Monitoring and, 135
  weight loss and, 232
sweets recipes
  Balsamic Berries, 303–4
  Butterfinger Bites, 309–10
  Chewy Oatmeal Chocolate Chip Cookies,
    312–13
  Chickpea Skillet Bars, 310–11
  Olive Oil Banana Bread, 304–5
  Protein Power Bites, 308–9
  Pumpkin Pie Parfaits, 305–7
"sweet tooth" flavors, 67–68

Taco Tuesday, revamping of, 63
Tangney, Christy, 8, 27, 39–40
tau tangles, levels of, 62
testes, DHA in, 21
TheOfficialMINDdiet.com, 134, 145, 178,
    181
thyroid issues, symptoms of, 15
time-based goals, 160
time management, 140
time-restricted eating, 176, 177
Toasted Nuts, 86, 321–22
tofu, 119, 219
trans fats, 23, *77,* 82, 117–21, *121*
traveling, tips for healthy eating, 157–59
triggers for eating, 58–59, 105, 215–16, 231
triglycerides, 110
Trust and Support
  as SMART MIND habit, 132, 165–67,
    201, *202*
  Week 1 and, 206
  Week 2 and, 211–12
  Week 3 and, 216–17
  Week 4 and, 221–22, 224

  Week 5 and, 227–28
  Week 6 and, 231–32
tryptophan, 90, 93
Turkey Chili, 262–63
Turkish Tabbouleh with Chicken Meatballs,
    95, 254–56
Tuscan Kale Salad, 293–94

U.S. POINTER (U.S. Study to Protect Brain
    Health through Lifestyle Intervention
    to Reduce Risk), 38, 39, 126
unsaturated fats
  as essential for brain health, 23–24
  extra-virgin olive oil (EVOO), 76, 77–83,
    105, 118, 119, 126, 154–55
  fat swaps, *121*
  as food category, 58, 76
  MIND Diet Targets, *78, 83*
  MIND Food Points, 76, *213*
  MIND Plate for Meal Planning and, 150,
    150, 151, *151,* 154–55
  nuts and seeds (Nut), 76, 83–87, 118, 121,
    154–55
  Week 3 and, 213–17
  weight loss and, 110
  whole grains and, 100

vascular dementia, 14
vegan diets, 23, 98, 132, 217
vegetable juices, 66
vegetable oils, hydrogenation of, 23, *77*
vegetables and fruit
  berries (Ber), *56,* 60, 72–75, 111, 112, 114,
    121, 153, 207
  as food category, 58, 60
  function of vegetables, 60–61
  leafy green vegetables (LG), *55,* 60, 61–64,
    207
  as low advanced glycation end products
    foods, 123
  MIND Diet Targets, *61, 65, 72*
  MIND Food Points, 60, *208*
  MIND Plate for Meal Planning and, 150,
    150, 151, *151,* 152–53, 154
  other vegetables (OV), *55,* 60, 64–71, 207
  Week 2 and, 207–12
  Week 3 and, 213
vegetarian diets, 91, 98, 132, 217
veggie bites, 66
Veggie Frittata, 174, 240–41
Veggie Hash with Eggs, 241–42
veggie scraps, 68–69, 81
veggie snacks, 67–68
Ventrelle, Jennifer, 8, 9, 33, 47–49
vitamin B, 90, 93, 100, 102, 106
vitamin B$_6$, 90, 106

vitamin B₁₂, 22–23, 90, 124
vitamin C, 72
vitamin D, 25, 124
vitamin deficiencies, 15
vitamin E, 20–21, 78, 80, 84, 100

waist size, 96
Warm Veggie Wrap, 285–86
water
  as beverage, 65, 159, 215–16
  in other vegetables, 65
  sugar swaps, 122
  weight loss and, 179, 229, 233
Wattles, Wallace D., 162
wearable technology, 167
weight loss
  alcohol consumption and, 115–16
  beans and legumes and, 107
  berries and, 73, 112
  body weight scale for, 170–71, 206, 212,
    216, 222
  calories and, 30, 61, 62, 65, 79, 86, 155,
    229, 232
  carbohydrates and, 103, 110–12
  extra-virgin olive oil and, 79, 83
  healthy food choices and, 175, 176
  intermittent fasting and, 175–78
  leafy green vegetables and, 61–62, 112
  lifestyle program or health coach for,
    179–81
  as long-term goal, 159
  long-term weight loss, 172–73, 233
  meal and snack frequency and, 174–75
  meal timing schedule, 173–79, 178, 222,
    223–24
  Mediterranean diet and, 40
  MIND Diet intervention trial and, 30, 35,
    41, 172
  nutrition tracking app for, 168–70, 171,
    206–7, 212, 216, 222, 233
  nuts and seeds and, 86
  other vegetables and, 65, 112
  physical activity and, 185, 188–89, 222,
    224
  proteins and, 96–98, 112
  repeated meals and, 178–79, 224
  Self-Monitoring and, 171, 172–73,
    212
  sleep and, 191
  tools for, 168–81
  Week 1 and, 206–7
  Week 2 and, 212
  Week 3 and, 216
  Week 4 and, 222–24
  Week 5 and, 228–29
  Week 6 and, 232
  weight loss maintenance strategies, 181
  weight loss targets and, 172–73, 207, 223,
    232, 233
weight management, 49, 59, 65, 73, 81–82,
  125
weight/strength training, 184, 186
White Fish with Olives and Artichokes, 90,
  275–77
white potatoes, 66
whole-grain breads, 102–3
whole-grain crackers, 105
whole-grain rice cakes, 104
whole grains (WG)
  carbohydrates and, 99–106, 110, 111, 123,
    153
  Foods to Choose list, 56
  as low advanced glycation end products
    foods, 123
  MIND Diet Target, *100*
  MIND Food Points, *111*, *225*
  servings versus portions of, 152
  shopping for, 101, *101*, 102–3
Willett, Walter, 18–19, 234
wine (Win)
  Foods to Choose list, *57*
  MIND Diet Target, *114*
  MIND Food Points and, 114–15, *115*, *225*
  moderate consumption of, 113–14, 121,
    225, 227, 229
Wing, Rena, 170

zeaxanthin, 35

About the Authors

Dr. Martha Clare Morris was a professor of epidemiology, the assistant provost for community research, and the director of the Rush Institute for Healthy Aging and the MIND Center for Brain Health at Rush University Medical Center in Chicago. She received her doctorate in epidemiology from the Harvard T.H. Chan School of Public Health and served as the principal investigator of multiple studies that investigate dietary risk factors for the development of Alzheimer's disease, cognitive decline, and other common chronic conditions of older people. Dr. Morris led a team of researchers at Rush University Medical Center to develop the MIND diet.

Laura Morris is a professionally trained chef, certified personal trainer, and certified nutrition consultant. She cowrote *Diet for the MIND* with Dr. Martha Clare Morris, and she has worked with a variety of age groups and special populations on the education and implementation of nutrition, food preparation, and exercise programs for healthy living.

Jennifer Ventrelle, MS, RDN, is a registered dietitian nutritionist certified in adult weight management, a certified personal trainer, and a mindfulness meditation teacher in the departments of Preventive Medicine and Clinical Nutrition at Rush University Medical Center. She was the lead dietitian on the MIND Diet Trial to Prevent Alzheimer's Disease and codirects the interventions for the U.S. POINTER Study, the largest clinical trial exploring the impact of lifestyle on cognitive decline in the United States. Ventrelle is the founder of CHOICE Nutrition and Wellness, LLC, partnering with individuals and organizations interested in integrative wellness and behavior change for mindful living.